PRESCRIPTION FOR HEALTH

*Living a Balanced Life
in a Toxic World*

Alan W. Gruning, DO, FACOEP

Faithful Life Publishers
North Fort Myers, FL

FaithfulLifePublishers.com

Prescription for Health

© 2015 by Alan W. Gruning, DO
ISBN: 978-1-63073-111-3

Published and printed by:
Faithful Life Publishers • North Fort Myers, FL 33903
888.720.0950 • info@FaithfulLifePublishers.com
www.FaithfulLifePublishers.com

Scripture quotations taken from the New American Standard Bible®, Copyright © 1960, 1962, 1963, 1968, 1971, 1972, 1973, 1975, 1977, 1995 by The Lockman Foundation. Used by permission. (www.Lockman.org)

All rights reserved. No part of this publication may be reproduced, stored in a retrieval system, or transmitted in any form or by any means—electronic, mechanical, photocopy, recording, or any other—except for brief quotations in printed review, without the prior permission of the author and/or publisher.

Printed in the United States of America

19 18 17 16 15   1 2 3 4 5

ABOUT THE AUTHOR

Alan W. Gruning, DO, FACOEP is Board Certified in Emergency Medicine and practiced that for 17 years, including 8 years as Medical Director. In 2001, he opened the International Center for Health and Wellness, a Christian medical practice, with offices in Fort Myers and Port Charlotte, Florida. He specializes in the care of acutely injured automobile accident patients. He also practices Functional Medicine, caring for those with complex disorders, including Fibromyalgia, Chronic Fatigue Syndrome, Autoimmune Disorders, and Environmental Toxicity, such as Biotoxin Illness, which other physicians have not been able to help.

Dr. Gruning is the founder of Christian Medical Ministries, operating the SW Florida Free Pain Clinic since 2010. Here, he cares for indigent patients with acute and chronic pain, without the use of medications, utilizing physical therapies, prayer, and the principles in this book. It is the only clinic of its kind in Florida. He previously was the founder of Christian Health Ministries, which provided free primary medical care to the poor in Charlotte County for 11 years.

Dr. Gruning is an accomplished and sought after teacher and speaker. He had his own television show on WRXY TV called Prescription for Health. He has taught in hospitals, EMS systems, and churches. An experienced Bible teacher, Dr. Gruning specializes in prophecy and discipleship. He speaks and preaches at churches in SW Florida. His passion is to educate the church and help the body of Christ to get healthy and fulfill God's purpose in the life of every follower of Jesus.

When not practicing medicine or teaching, Dr. Gruning serves as an online Chat Coach for the Search for Jesus team, an internet evangelism ministry of the Billy Graham Evangelistic Association. He gets to chat with seekers from all over the world about Jesus and helps them find Christ over the internet.

Alan and his wife, Janet, have been married since 1983. Janet is his practice manager and partner in ministry. They have two grown children, Lauren and Christopher, and two grandchildren, Tyler and Bethany.

DEDICATION

This book is dedicated to all those who are struggling with pain, fatigue, digestive problems and mental fog and have been told there is nothing wrong with them and they must be depressed and needed pills. You are not mentally ill. There is something physically wrong with you. But, not for much longer. You will get better and you will fulfill the purpose the Lord has for your life.

ACKNOWLEDGMENTS

Thank you to my wife Janet for putting up with all my Big Dreams, being the voice of practical wisdom in my life and loving me unconditionally.

Thank you to my daughter, Lauren Thomas, for her invaluable help transcribing my ramblings. I am so proud of the woman of God, wife and mother she has become.

Thank you to my son, Christopher, for his eye for detail and his ability to find the right words. I am so proud of the man of God he has become.

Thank you to all those patients and staff who encouraged me to write this book.

Thank You to the Holy Spirit for inspiring me to write this book when I had a block and did not know how to proceed.

Thank You to my Lord and Savior, Jesus Christ, for choosing to use a sinner like me in His ministries.

TABLE OF CONTENTS

Introduction 1

1. My Journey into Holistic Health 7
2. The Problems 15
3. Is There a Conspiracy? 29
4. The Bottom Line 35
5. Our Toxic World 51
6. Your Prescription for Health 77
7. Eat to Live! 83
8. Don't Live to Eat! 109
9. I Can't Sleep 139
10. Eliminating the Toxins 155
11. Vitamins and Supplements for Health 167
12. Supporting Your Endocrine System 197
13. Detoxification Made Simple? 213
14. The Final Key to Holistic Health 221
Appendix 1 — God's Promises for You 227

INTRODUCTION

This could be one of the most important books you have ever read. Or, it could be a tremendous waste of your time. The choice is yours. It all depends on your attitude going in.

For years my patients and staff have been encouraging me to write a book about what I tell my patients to do and how I try to live. Honestly, I did not think I had the time or patience to do it. However, as I began to look at the state of health in America, and especially in the church, I knew that the time to write this book was now.

I prayed for the Lord to show me about the need for this book and to speak to me about when to write it. Recently, I felt the Lord impressing on me that the time to sit down and write it had come and that I had His blessing to do it. I knew that without the inspiration of the Holy Spirit, this would just be a collection of words and ideas. I want to see the lives and health of people in America, and the church, change for the better. Words by themselves won't do that.

Much of what you are going to read is not new information. Sometimes we have all the information we need to know, but it is just how it is organized and presented that makes the difference. That is not to say that I don't have some special new revelations for you, but I think the big thing I can do for you is try to make all of this very practical and something you can implement in your life and the lives of your family.

There is a lot at stake. Every indication is that despite all of our money spent on the most expensive and elaborate health care system in the world, the health of the American people is worse than ever. If nothing changes, we are heading for a national disaster, not from some external enemy or a natural catastrophe, but from within our own nation. And unless you do something to change things and help yourself and your family, I don't believe our government and its myriad bureaucratic agencies will ever change things enough to make a difference for your health.

Much of this book came from the inspiration of doing my own TV show and the feedback I have received from patients and viewers. *Prescription for Health* aired on WRXY TV for the last 6 months of 2012. You can still see the shows on my YouTube channel. Unfortunately, it had to come to an end due to a lack of finances. I am very appreciative of the sponsors who helped me put it on the air for a time. Who knows, someday I may do TV again.

For now, I believe God wants me to teach the American people, and particularly the body of Christ, how to live a balanced life in a toxic world. As I speak with pastors and church leaders, it is clear that one of the big problems we are facing is a population of church leaders and churchgoers who are sick-physically, emotionally, and spiritually. This sickness is affecting how people are able to serve and be involved in church life and ministry. The most common complaint is that of fatigue and just not feeling well enough to do things. It is hard to get motivated to serve the Lord when you feel terrible most of the time.

Fatigue.

That is what physicians hear a lot from patients. It is one of the most common complaints in physician offices. The basic blood tests are normal and no obvious cause is found. The numbers have been already treated with prescription medications. In a busy medical practice, the patient is told that they must be depressed and are prescribed antidepressants or referred to a psychiatrist. Or they may be told they are not getting enough sleep and prescribed a sleeping pill. Or they may be told they are anxious and prescribed an anti-anxiety pill or referred to a psychiatrist for that. Any way you look at it, the cause is not found and the patients are simply not believed. The path of least resistance for most physician practices is referral to the psychiatric or psychological specialist.

But what if there are causes for this fatigue and not feeling well? The problem may not be identified by the usual blood tests done by most physicians, but that does not mean the problem is all in our heads. Certainly there are a lot of pharmaceutical companies making a lot of money from those decisions. Since they are the ones sponsoring most of the Continuing Education programs we physicians attend, it is understandable how that can happen. In fact, to believe and practice anything different than the party line leads to accusations of not practicing according to the standard of care.

There are many causes for fatigue and why we are not feeling well. There are reasons why Americans are sicker than ever with little hope of things getting better. In fact, every indication is that things will get much worse. We are going to look at the causes and solutions and what you can do to change all of this. Along the way, I hope that you will feel better and that a myriad of chronic diseases will be prevented. Then I hope you will go out and give back to others, educating them and getting involved in ministries to serve others, especially the sick and impoverished.

Where do we start? I call these my 4 F's.

Fresh Start.

You need to forget about all those past failed attempts to get healthy, lose weight, and change your life. This will be totally different. You are not doing this alone. You will have a lot of guidance from me. Don't live in the past. Look forward to a healthy future. You will not fail this time.

Facts.

Forget about past misinformation you were given. Fad diets, crazy detoxifications, and expensive supplements won't get you where you want to be. I will give you the facts needed to see the real issues involved and to make the right decisions to live a healthy, balanced life so you can better serve your family, church and community.

Faith.

You must have some measure of faith that you will be able to do this. Not only will you have a lot of help from me, but also you will have the help of our mighty God Who wants you to have an abundant life on this earth. He promised in Jeremiah 29:11, *'For I know the plans that I have for you,' declares the Lord, 'plans for welfare and not for calamity to give you a future and a hope.*

Fellowship.

There is strength in community. I encourage you to take this journey together with a few people. Perhaps study this with a spouse, sibling, friend, small group at church, or your co-workers. Accountability is important. And you will be already helping others to get healthy while you pursue a healthier lifestyle.

Here is a warning. To do nothing is to do something. Don't expect things to change unless you change them. To continue to do the same things over and over and to expect different results is Einstein's definition of insanity. Don't be insane. Make the changes needed to get healthy and stay healthy.

In this book, I will not be citing lots of peer reviewed journals and scientific articles. Trust me, I have already done the research, but the amount of information out there is overwhelming. The literature coming out about nutrition, supplements and other natural health treatments is staggering and our understanding is changing daily. By the time you read this, much of the articles I could cite would be obsolete. However, I will give you my opinions and synthesis of the knowledge available at the time of this writing to guide you into sound decisions for your health. Along the way, I will reference some significant sources of information that you can investigate yourself and keep up on what is being discovered in the areas of nutrition, toxins and health.

My advice to you is to keep up with what is going on in research and don't listen to every new story that comes out on the TV or the internet. You have to embark upon a life of learning and growing as knowledge is changing so fast that it is nearly impossible to stay current.

Several good organizations can help you keep up with what is going on and have magazines/websites to help. Examples include Environmental Working Group, Institute for Responsible Technology, Surviving Mold, and Life Extension Foundation. I also have respect for Dr. Oz and how he is willing to go against the traditional medical establishment to bring people the truth.

Throughout this book you will see **PFH Action Points** to help summarize important concepts and direct you to take specific steps. I hope these will be your "baby steps" to get started on your journey to better health. You can then add to that with more information from this book to fine-tune your approach to getting your life back in balance.

The Bible says in 1 Corinthians 6:19-20, *Or do you not know that your body is a temple of the Holy Spirit who is in you, whom you have from God, and that you are not your own? For you have been bought with a price: therefore glorify God in your body.* While this was written specifically about sexual immorality, it is easy to extend this verse into every area of our life, including our health. If we keep doing things that we know are hurting our bodies, are we really bringing God the glory He is due? I don't know about you, but if the Holy Spirit of God is living in me, I want to make sure that His home is in the best condition possible!

PFH Action Point

- **Overview of *Prescription for Health: Living a Balanced Life in a Toxic World***
- **Identify the problems we are facing in healthcare as a nation**
- **Identify the individual challenges to your health and the health of your family**
- **Present a detailed, comprehensive treatment plan with practical guidelines for you to implement now**
- **Restore the balance to your body, mind and spirit**
- **Experience a better quality of life, not just a longer life**

Chapter 1
MY JOURNEY INTO HOLISTIC HEALTH

There I was, sitting in the office of the hospital's Chief Operating Officer. I had been there many times in the past, in my position as Medical Director of the Emergency Care Center. However, I had stepped down from that position a few years earlier. And things were different now. The COO, and then eventual hospital president I had worked with for many years, Steve, had left. Now a new administration was in place. For me to be here, there must be a problem.

I reflected back on the past. I had devoted my life to Emergency Medicine. Ever since I was a child that was all I knew I had wanted to do. Being a doctor, then an Emergency Medicine specialist, had been my dream. I had been able to live out that dream for 17 years and had even diversified into Emergency Department administration as my hospital had recognized my leadership abilities. However, the life span of most emergency physicians is limited. Most burn out within 10 years. I had exceeded the average, but I knew that my days in the ED were going to come to an end.

In preparation for a transition out of Emergency Medicine, I had taken extra training and become certified in Occupational and Preventive Medicine. Steve had asked me if I wanted to help open up an Occupational Medicine clinic to care for Workers Comp injuries. I thought it was a logical progression for me. So, with the hospital's help, I was heading up a program off site with a wonderful staff and having a great time caring for injured workers. I was getting to develop relationships with patients, something that was very foreign to me as an ED physician. The ED life is one of brief patient interactions and much stress, including changing from day to night shifts often, which was taking its toll on me.

I thought things were going pretty well. My physician partners were assuming more of the administrative functions and we had brought in another physician to help with the shifts that I was cutting back on. I was spending more time with my family and pursuing some other things that were important to me. However, there was trouble in paradise. Little did I know that this meeting would change the entire direction of my life.

The COO addressed me very matter of fact, telling me that she had heard that I was praying with patients and talking to them about Jesus. I told her that was true, that I was offering to pray with patients if they desired and was talking with those who wanted to know more about Jesus and my relationship with Him. Odd, I thought, because this had never been a problem with Steve. I had been very open with him about my spiritual life and my desire to merge faith with medicine. It was a topic that was just starting to be openly discussed back in 2001, and several medical schools were incorporating this subject into their curriculum, in a general way. All of the studies showed that patients wanted to discuss their spiritual needs with their physician, but that none have ever asked them. I was just doing what the patients desired, good customer satisfaction. Steve had given me his blessing, as long as he did not hear any complaints from patients. It had been thrilling for both of us that there were not any complaints, only compliments for the caring environment in our clinic and in the ER when I was on duty.

I'll never forget what the COO told me. She said I had to stop offering to pray with patients and speaking to patients about Jesus, as it was the job of the clergy on staff and not part of my job description. I needed to call for a pastoral consult when someone wanted to discuss his or her spiritual life or pray. I informed her that was impractical as the pastoral care was done by one person, a former pastor, and he was not always immediately available for someone to pray with or ask spiritual questions. What was wrong with me meeting that need?

She responded that faith and medicine have no place together and she needed me to just provide their medical care, not address any spiritual needs. I was totally floored by her response. This was certainly contrary to what was emerging in medicine and certainly violated my rights to practice my religion in a free nation. I explained to her that as a Christian it is part of my religious beliefs to bring Jesus into the workplace or whatever environment I find myself and meet the spiritual needs of people, wherever they may be at the time. This included the hospital, my occupational medicine clinic, my free medical clinic, the store, or wherever I happened to be.

What she said next is typical of what is happening in medicine, but also in America in general. She said that she was also a Christian and understood that what she does on Sunday morning has nothing to do with what happens the rest of the week. In other words, there is to be no mixing of secular and sacred. Well, if that is true, we should just throw out a lot of the Bible, especially the New Testament, where the writers go to great lengths to help us understand how to integrate the Christian life with whatever we are doing, whether it is work, family, church, or recreation. I now understand that this is the definition of a fan of Jesus, not a follower of Jesus.

I explained to the COO that I had a different view and took my marching orders from Jesus, Who made it very clear that I was to go into all the world and make disciples. That included my workplace. I would not stop offering to pray with patients or staff (many of whom would come to me with their needs) and I would not stop offering Jesus to people. There is ultimately only one underlying cause for all human misery, and that is sin. There is only one cure for sin, and that is Jesus Christ and the cross. To not offer that to people would be like withholding life-saving treatment from a dying patient.

I had drawn a line in the sand. I thought to myself that this is what it means to be persecuted for your faith. No, I was not living in some Muslim country where I was being told to deny Jesus as my Savior and

Lord or I would be killed. But, I was having to take a stand for Jesus and religious freedom that so many of our brave service men and women paid the ultimate price for. I was not going to back down, no matter what it meant.

She said that if I persisted in what I was doing, she would be forced to terminate the contract for our Emergency Physician Group and my services as head of the Occupational Medicine program. Well, there it was. Decision time. No turning back. It was time to put up or shut up. It was one thing to threaten me, but to threaten my whole physician group, that was another matter. I told her that I would let her know my decision and left.

I knew I could not continue to practice medicine under her rules. However, there were huge implications if I were to leave. I had a no-compete clause, so if I decided to stay in Emergency Medicine, it would mean traveling to the next city. There would be financial uncertainties for my family. But, to stay and live under the COO's conditions was unthinkable. I thought about going over her head to some of the other power brokers on the hospital board I knew very well, but ultimately did not think I would get much support on this issue. It was only important to me.

As I went into the ED after the meeting, I saw Sheri sitting at our physician desk. She was an Advanced Registered Nurse Practitioner (ARNP) and a good friend. We loved working together. She was a solid Christian and was always a calm in the storm.

I remembered when I was driving to work in 1997 and I asked God what He wanted me to do for Him. I had become convinced we were living in the last days. I was an ardent student of prophecy and understood the signs of the times Jesus had spoken about. I knew it was all happening just the way the Bible had said and that time was short for me to accomplish whatever He had planned for me. I heard God's voice in the car. I am not sure if it was audible or just in my head. But it was very clear, like He was right there speaking to me.

The Lord told me He wanted me to take care of the poor. Well, that was pretty general. How did He want me to do that? So, I asked Him out loud what He wanted me to do. This idea materialized in my head of a free medical clinic that merged physical, emotional and spiritual healing. But, how would all that come together?

I got to the ED and Sheri was there. I sat down at our desk and told her what God had just said to me. Her response was very calm and assured. She said that if the Lord was in it, He would make it happen. I did not need to know how or when, but it would happen. Not two minutes later, the ED Secretary on duty came in and said that the President of the Medical Society was there to meet me. Funny, I thought, I did not have any appointments that morning, as I usually don't schedule any while I am on duty.

Pat came in and asked me to do a lecture for the medical society meeting in a few months. I said I would. Then, I felt like I should ask her something. I told her I had a crazy idea of starting a free medical clinic and did not know where to begin. She said it was not a crazy idea and that she could and would love to help me do it. Sheri looked at me with that "I told you so" look. The rest is history. Christian Health Ministries was born in a few months and cared for the poor of Charlotte County for 11 years.

I sat down this day and told Sheri of my conversation with the COO. Again, she was very calm and seemed absolutely sure of what she was going to say next. I do believe God talks through people today, just like He did with the prophets of old. She said that I should open up my own medical practice. The thought had not even crossed my mind. Open my own practice? It would certainly solve a lot of problems. I could stay locally and practice medicine the way God wanted me to. But, how would all that happen? It was almost impossible to start a solo medical practice from scratch without help from some hospital or big entity.

Again, Sheri was very matter of fact with me. She said that if God was in it, then it would happen. I asked my wife Janet, and while she had some reservations about radically changing our lives and the lives of our children, she was very supportive of whatever the Lord had laid on my heart. She was my rock who God used to lead me to Jesus in the first place. Well, by way of many miracles that I don't have the time to go into detail about right now, I left the hospital, saving my physician group, and opened my own medical practice. I dedicated it as a ministry to the Lord and made a covenant with Jesus that I would care for people physically, emotionally and spiritually. We eventually opened two offices, one in Port Charlotte and one in Fort Myers.

My initial goal was to care for two groups of patients that the Lord had spoken to me about that were not getting the best care because most doctors did not want them in their practice: auto accident patients and workers compensation patients. Our offices were set up to provide comprehensive care for them. Along the way, we started to provide some primary care as patients begged us to see them, especially former hospital employees.

I remember in early 2004 I started to feel very bad. I was exhausted and barely able to get through my day. My staff was concerned. I was not thinking as clearly as normal and my staff had to keep me awake. I remember that there were times I was falling asleep while talking to patients, not a good thing for a caring physician to do. I thought I had a virus, since that is what we say when we don't know what is wrong with someone. However, it did not run its course and the fatigue persisted.

I did the usual lab tests on myself, but they were normal. I went to a few of my physician friends and they could not find anything wrong with me. Was I depressed, stressed, or overworked? That was the usual answer for most of us practicing traditional medicine. But I knew that none of those were the cause. There was something wrong, but I did not know what it was or how to treat it. I know now that I had the symptoms of Chronic Fatigue Syndrome.

At that time, my Nurse Practitioner, Mary Louise, told me about a speaker at a conference she had been to recently. He was a holistic physician who spoke about natural treatment of thyroid disease. She had one of his books and asked if I wanted to read it since it made a lot of sense to her. I was desperate, so I reluctantly took the book. So began a journey that would radically change my life and the way I practiced medicine forever.

Since that time, a lot has happened. Hurricane Charley struck Punta Gorda, Florida and we lost our home (with us in it) and our Port Charlotte office, causing us to move to Fort Myers; our office and home were eventually rebuilt. Financial struggles became a way of life for us in a changing medical environment. Employee changes became a recurring nightmare as people left to go where God wanted them and we had to find the right people to replace them. However, through it all, the Lord has been with my family, our ministry, and me. He has taught me a lot and I am learning more all the time. He is using our ministry and me in incredible ways to help a lot of patients, including pastors and missionaries.

Currently, I practice Holistic Complimentary Medicine, combining the best of traditional medicine with natural therapies that heal. Since I seek to treat the cause of sickness and disease, rather than the symptoms, and restore balance to the whole person, I fit into the emerging field called Functional Medicine. I don't consider myself an Alternative Medicine Practitioner since I don't believe that many of these belief systems are consistent with my Christian beliefs and many of the treatments have no scientific basis. I am open-minded, but I see no evidence of a life energy field that can purportedly be manipulated by these practitioners. I have had numerous well-meaning Christians tell me that this life energy is just another name for the Holy Spirit. My Bible says that the Holy Spirit is part of the Triune Godhead and lives only in followers of Jesus Christ. He is not an energy field, but a spiritual Being. We can't manipulate the Holy Spirit; He is supposed to be our Teacher, Counselor, Comforter and Helper.

Besides acutely injured auto accident patients, I see patients with Fibromyalgia, Chronic Fatigue and Immune Dysfunction Syndrome (now being called Systemic Exertion Intolerance Disease), Autoimmune Disorders, Hormone Imbalances, and Environmental Toxicity. I also see patients in our free medical clinic weekly, many of which are dealing with the same issues as my office patients, but without the medical coverage or finances to deal with them. Gleaning from my comprehensive treatment regimen for these very sick people over the years, I have a lot of things I want to share with you to help you get well and stay that way.

Let's get started.

Chapter 2
THE PROBLEMS

In this section, we will identify the problems we are facing in healthcare as a nation. We will also look at the individual challenges to your health and the health of your family.

We are facing a health crisis in this country of unprecedented proportions. No, I am not talking about the health care crisis. That is a different, but related issue. Certainly the poor health of our population has precipitated the rapidly escalating costs that our government is trying to come to grips with. We spend more on health care than almost every other industrialized nation. Why are we in such a crisis then?

Throwing more money at our health problems is not solving it. More technology and prescriptions are not solving it. More health care providers and facilities are not solving it. More government intervention, laws and bureaucracy are not and will not solve it. Education programs will not solve it as long as they are teaching the wrong things.

The solution for the health crisis is much more basic. It involves individuals making the right decisions about how they live their lives. Not because someone tells them they have to, but because they want to. And it involves providing people with the knowledge and tools they need to make responsible, educated decisions.

I remember when I first started getting involved with the American Heart Association, teaching Basic Life Support. This goes way back, to the mid 1970's. I remember that at that time the statistics were that about 650,000 people died in this country each year of heart disease. Guess what? 2013 statistics show that 600,000 people die of heart disease each year. Not much difference. 40 years, trillions of dollars, all of that education provided to physicians and the population on risk factor modification, lots of government programs, untold numbers of prescriptions for statins and other drugs that we were told would reduce heart disease mortality and morbidity, millions of surgical procedures like stents and bypass, and what is there to show for it? Something is terribly wrong.

Sure, there has been some progress. The anti-smoking message got out and less people smoke. The ridiculous commercials glorifying and promoting tobacco use have ceased. However, they have been replaced with endless commercials glorifying alcohol in all its forms. More people drink than ever, despite all the evidence detailing how it destroys our bodies and destroys families.

And what about cancer? Is there any less of that? No. What about diabetes? It is exploding as the obesity epidemic progresses. Americans are getting bigger each year with no end in sight. What about thyroid disease? It is increasing at exponential rates. Why? What about Autoimmune Diseases? They are increasing rapidly, and it is not because of better detection.

It is not just chronic diseases that are at issue. People just don't feel well. Yes, some of it is that they are obese and carrying a lot of extra weight. But fatigue is a major problem, one of the most common complaints in a physician's office. Fatigue is robbing Americans of productivity and happiness. It is costing the health care system enormous resources to evaluate and treat fatigue complaints. It is costing business and industry enormous amounts of time and money. It is costing the church, too: members and pastors feel unable to serve in ministry to their full potential because they feel exhausted. So the quality of our lives is deteriorating even if our life span is not.

I don't want to burden you with a bunch of statistics. We all know we are in a deep mess. That is probably why you have decided to read this book. However, a few statistics are very revealing.

Let's look at obesity first, since a lot of other diseases stem from this issue. Using BMI (Body Mass Index) of 25-30 as overweight and over

30 as obese, more than 1/3 of adults and 17% of children/adolescents are obese in the U.S. About one third of adults are overweight. Thus, 2/3 of the US adult population is above their ideal body weight. Men and women are equally obese. Adults aged 60 and over are more likely to be obese than younger adults. 12 states have an obesity prevalence of over 30% (Mississippi is 34%).

A recent study, published by Life Extension, shows the BMI to be inaccurate, especially in women. Serum Leptin levels and measurement of body fat appear to be more accurate. Using these measures, the obesity epidemic is even greater than our government is telling us.

What should we weigh? According to the Metropolitan Life Insurance Company Height/Weight Charts of 1983, probably a lot less than we think. I am about 6 feet tall (although I am shrinking a little) and a medium frame (although I envision myself more muscular). According to these charts, I should weigh 157-170 lbs. Currently, I weigh 165. I have worked hard to get there. I feel better when I weigh 165. The thing about these charts, which you can search for easily on the internet and I have reproduced on the next page, is that they should not change over time. Just because we think it is fine to be bigger and weigh more does not mean it is healthy. There was a time in our nation when people weighed a lot less and felt a lot better.

So, what is the big deal if we weigh a little more? Well, besides not fitting into the clothes you used to be able to wear and having to spend a lot of extra money buying new clothes, there are clearly a number of health effects due to obesity. These include coronary heart disease, Type 2 Diabetes, cancers (endometrial, breast, and colon), hypertension, Peripheral Vascular Disease, stroke, liver and gall bladder disease, sleep apnea and respiratory diseases, osteoarthritis, hormonal imbalances, abnormal menses, and infertility. Looking at this list, it is clear that a lot of our current national health problems are due to our increasing weight. It is also clear that large portions of our health care expenditures are due to our increasing weight. If you want to fix the health care crisis, the people of this nation must lose weight.

What Should We Weigh?

Metropolitan Life Insurance Company Height/Weight Charts, 1983

MEN	SMALL FRAME	MEDIUM FRAME	LARGE FRAME
5' 2"	128-134	131-141	138-150
5' 3"	130-136	133-143	140-153
5' 4"	132-138	135-145	142-156
5' 5"	134-140	137-148	144-160
5' 6"	136-142	139-151	146-164
5' 7"	138-145	142-154	149-168
5' 8"	140-148	145-157	152-172
5' 9"	142-151	148-160	155-176
5' 10"	144-154	151-163	158-180
5' 11"	146-157	154-166	161-184
6' 0"	149-160	157-170	164-188
6' 1"	152-164	160-174	168-192
6' 2"	155-168	164-178	172-197
6' 3"	158-172	167-182	176-202
6' 4"	162-176	171-187	181-207

Weights at ages 25-59 based on lowest mortality. Weight in pounds according to frame (in indoor clothing weighing 5 lbs., shoes with 1" heels)

WOMEN	SMALL FRAME	MEDIUM FRAME	LARGE FRAME
4' 10"	102-111	109-121	118-131
4' 11"	103-113	111-123	120-134
5' 0"	104-115	113-126	122-137
5' 1"	106-118	115-129	125-140
5' 2"	108-121	118-132	128-143
5' 3"	111-124	121-135	131-147
5' 4"	114-127	124-138	134-151
5' 5"	117-130	127-141	137-155
5' 6"	120-133	130-144	140-159
5' 7"	123-136	133-147	143-163
5' 8"	126-139	136-150	146-167
5' 9"	129-142	139-153	149-170
5' 10"	132-145	142-156	152-173
5' 11"	135-148	145-159	155-176
6' 0"	138-151	148-162	158-179

Weights at ages 25-59 based on lowest mortality. Weight in pounds according to frame (in indoor clothing weighing 3 lbs., shoes with 1" heels)

What are the causes of this obesity epidemic? We will be looking at these in detail later. For now, understand that this is a complex problem with many causes. Wheat, High Fructose Corn Syrup, sugar-sweetened beverages, fast food, and diet sodas/food are certainly some of the biggest culprits. Endocrine Disruptors such as plastics, pesticides, and heavy metals have poisoned our metabolism and disrupted the balance in our bodies. thyroid, adrenal, and hormone imbalances have affected our metabolism and body structure. Stress and sleep deprivation have also contributed to the problem. As you can see, to fix the obesity problem, we have to fix a lot of other things first.

Related to this obesity epidemic is an epidemic of Metabolic Syndrome. It affects 47 million Americans (1 out of 6 people). According to the American Heart Association and the National Heart, Lung, and Blood Institute, Metabolic Syndrome is present if you have three or more of the following signs:

- Blood pressure equal to or higher than 130/85 mmHg
- Fasting blood sugar (glucose) higher than 99 mg/dL
- Large waist circumference (length around the waist): Men - 40 inches or more; Women - 35 inches or more
- Low HDL cholesterol: Men - under 40 mg/dL; Women - under 50 mg/dL
- Triglycerides equal to or higher than 150 mg/dL

Metabolic Syndrome increases the risk of coronary artery disease, stroke, and Type 2 Diabetes dramatically. Note that LDL cholesterol is not on this list. We'll talk about all the misinformation we have received about LDL cholesterol later.

Diabetes is at epidemic numbers and is growing at an alarming rate. When I was growing up, we only heard rarely about someone having diabetes. Now, it is accepted as a normal part of getting older. However, it is affecting a lot of young people, too. Diabetes affects over 29 million Americans with 89 million meeting the criteria for pre-diabetes and at risk for developing diabetes in the near future (and probably will). 1 in 3 people born in the U.S. in 2000 will develop diabetes during their lifetime if trends continue. The lifetime risk numbers are actually 33% for men and 39% for women. The risk is higher for African Americans and Hispanics (1 in 2 for Hispanic girls and women!). Complications of diabetes include heart and vascular disease, renal failure, blindness and other eye diseases, neuropathy, and amputation.

It is interesting that more and more studies are coming out confirming what Functional Medicine specialists have been saying all along. That lifestyle changes reduce the risk of diabetes and actually can cure it. The DaQing study in China showed that a combination of diet and exercise reduced diabetes by 42%. The Finnish Diabetes Prevention Study showed that lifestyle changes reduced diabetes by 58%. The US Diabetes Prevention Program published their 10 year follow up results in Lancet and showed that at 4 years into the trial, lifestyle changes reduced diabetes by 58% and at 10 years by 34%. Apparently, many stopped their lifestyle changes and resorted back to their diabetic state after 4 years. These results were far better than for Metformin, the gold standard drug used for comparisons. What do all these studies indicate? Lifestyle changes prevent and reverse diabetes for up to half of patients. What has not been taken into account in these studies is the presence of toxins. We will look at how toxins cause and contribute to diabetes later.

Mention the word *cancer*, and fear will explode in the minds of most of us. Cancer seems to be increasing at an alarming rate. It is not that we just hear about it more than when I was growing up. There will be 1.6 million new cases of cancer in the U.S. this year (excluding skin cancers). This cancer will result in 580,000 deaths this year (1500/day). The most common cancers are lung, prostate and colorectal in men and lung, breast and colorectal in women. The lifetime probability of being diagnosed with an invasive cancer is 45% for men and 38% for women. What is causing this explosion in cancers? The answers are many and varied. We will examine some of them.

Cardiovascular Disease is a category that includes Heart Disease, Hypertension, and Peripheral Vascular Disease. It is the leading cause of death in the U.S., killing 600,000 Americans annually. Stroke is the 4th leading cause. 76 million adults are hypertensive, with many being poorly controlled. What is contributing to these numbers? We already mentioned that smoking has declined; yet 21% of men and 17.5% of women over 18 are smokers. 20% of boys and 19% of girls in grades 9-12 are smokers. There is a lot more work to be done to combat this known killer of our people, tobacco use.

72% of men and 62% of women are overweight or obese; 32% of boys and 31% of girls are overweight or obese. There is a direct correlation with between weight and Cardiovascular Disease risk. Less than 1% of U.S. adults meet the definition for the Ideal Healthy Diet; no children meet that goal. Only 20% of adults and 37% of 9-12 graders meet federal guidelines for physical activity. There is also a direct correlation between physical activity levels and Cardiovascular Disease. We have a lot of work to do with weight loss and physical activity levels if we intend to make a dent on these numbers.

What about medical errors? No one likes to discuss this, but it is a very significant cause of death and disability in our country. Studies seem to indicate that medical errors cause around 200,000 deaths in the US each year! That makes it one of the highest causes of death and does not routinely show up in statistics you will see. These errors include giving the wrong medication or using the wrong dose. Many are now caused by errors in using the electronic record systems, that doctors and hospitals have been forced into using, and the inability to correctly read doctor's orders. Many of these errors occur in hospitals and nursing homes. There are also errors in correctly diagnosing and treating diseases in a timely manner, when patients can still be helped. In addition, there is the risk when admitted to the hospital or nursing facility of acquiring a deadly super bug infection, resistant to treatment. The bottom line is to try to avoid these errors by staying healthy through prevention.

PFH Action Point
- **Obesity is a worldwide health epidemic, affecting young and old**
- **Metabolic Syndrome and diabetes are near epidemic levels**
- **Cancer seems to affect every family**

- **Cardiovascular disease is still the leading cause of death in the U.S.**
- **Medical errors cause much death and disability**

Thyroid disease is another problem that is exploding in this country. When I first started out in medicine, thyroid problems were some of those rare issues we would deal with as a specialist. Now, everyone seems to have it. Most thyroid disorders are undiagnosed. The incidence might be up to 30% of U.S. adults. Officially 20 million or 7.3% Americans have thyroid diseases, the most common being Hypothyroidism. Most thyroid disease patients are misdiagnosed as fatigue, fibromyalgia, chronic fatigue, depression, arthritis, allergies, and obesity; as you can see, it can look like a lot of things. Thyroid problems can result in immune dysfunction, weight issues, hormonal imbalances, osteoporosis, heart failure, dysrhthmias, and a host of GI problems. It may also be a cause of some cancers.

Autoimmune diseases are also exploding in our nation. This is where the body attacks its own organs and tissues, thinking they are a foreign invader. Examples of autoimmune disorders include Hashimoto's (Autoimmune) Thyroiditis, Grave's Disease, Multiple Sclerosis, Psoriasis, Rheumatoid Arthritis, Crohn's Disease, Ulcerative Colitis, Systemic Lupus, Celiac Disease, Myasthenia Gravis, and a host of other illnesses. Again, these things were rare a few decades ago; now, physicians are all expected to know about them. I deal a lot with autoimmune and thyroid diseases in my practice. We'll talk more about where they come from later.

Anxiety and depression are the most common complaints at a family doctor's office today. It seems like everyone is on something because they are anxious or depressed. In fact 18% of adults and 30% of young people suffer from Anxiety Disorder. We live in an era of information overload, which is directly contributing to these problems. Between the TV and the internet, social media, smart phones and tablets we are bombarded with slick marketing to tell us we are all sick and need a pill to fix it. The majority of people want a pill for their problems; they don't think they have the time or money for counseling. Just look at all the TV commercials for prescription drugs; it sure looks like we are all sick and need to be on something to make us feel better. By the way, have you seen these ads? 25% of the time is spent on the problem the drug will supposedly fix and 75% on the potential side effects of the drug, including coma and death.

Related to this is the topic of Bipolar Illness. What was a rare diagnosis a decade ago now seems to be commonplace. Do all of these people really have Bipolar Illness and need a drug to help them? These drugs are potentially very dangerous and toxic. The advertisements also tell us that if one drug is not enough, you may need a second one!

Is all of this mental illness a physical, emotional, or spiritual issue? It may be all three. Physical illness and imbalance, accompanied by emotional fatigue and stress, and a lack of spiritual life and a relationship with God may all be responsible. Clearly pharmaceuticals do not fix all of that. However, companies are making a lot of money telling you they can!

Let's talk about fatigue for a moment. Fatigue is one of the most common presenting complaints at your family doctor's office. The information obtained in a typical primary care ten-minute office visit and the screening lab studies ordered does not usually identify the cause. So, the symptoms are treated with, you guessed it, prescription drugs. It is easy for the health care provider and expected by the patient. They are band-aids on a much deeper problem that no one, including the patient, seems to want to address. Often, these band-aids are psych drugs, like antidepressants and anti-anxiety agents, or sleep meds.

Fatigue is robbing Americans of their productivity and happiness. It is costing the health care system billions of dollars to evaluate and treat this collection of disorders. It is costing businesses billions in lost time, productivity, and insurance costs. Fatigue is costing the church members who are too exhausted to attend or be involved in its ministries. It is also costing the church pastors and their wives who are too ill to continue on in ministry. I know, because I see them.

Pain is the latest hot topic. Everyone is in pain, it seems, and needs pain pills. Short acting, long acting, from the pharmacy or from the streets, the abuse of pain pills is a huge problem. I live in Florida. We were the worst state in the nation for pill mills, places where people could come and pay cash for an "office visit" and get large prescriptions for controlled substances, typically narcotics. People came from all over the US to get their drugs here. We had to swallow some pretty tough laws and rules in Florida to rein this all in. And the ones who are suffering are the legitimate patients with pain who can't find a doctor to prescribe what they need for fear of the DEA coming down on them.

Don't get me wrong. I deal with acutely injured auto accident patients and very sick people with Fibromyalgia. There are legitimate patients who need help with their pain. Whether it is a cancer patient or someone with failed back surgery, patients with real pain deserve real treatment. However, we don't need a pain pill for everything. Yes, I have prescribed hundreds of short acting narcotics to patients with injuries and surgical procedures that needed temporary help with their pain. But how did we get in the mess we are in with pill mills and pain meds being the most abused drugs in America, responsible for many of the deadly overdoses we see? Are people really in this much pain, more so than at other times in our history?

Pain is a complex sensation. It is not just the physical insult that causes pain. The perception of pain is affected by many variables, including nutritional status, hydration, sleep deprivation, emotional state, stress, medications, and toxins. So, there is not only an underlying cause to most pain, but factors that affect how we perceive it. What if those factors are the same things that are making us sick in general? If that is true, then we can reduce the number of patients with pain, and the severity of their pain, with lifestyle changes. We'll be looking at those changes shortly.

Americans are sleep deprived, too. I speak to patients every day that can't sleep for various reasons. Either they can't get to sleep, because they can't turn off their brain or they get a second wind at night, or they can't stay asleep, waking up many times and not being able to fall back asleep for hours. These are exhausted people, physically and emotionally. It takes a toll on their productivity at work and their relationships at home. They don't have the capacity to deal with problems and stressors anymore. They fall asleep driving or their reaction times are impaired, just like someone drinking alcohol. They are just trying to get through each day, often resorting to energy drinks and other stimulants to keep going. It is termed Excessive Daytime Sedation (EDS) and it is a recipe for disaster.

As of the early 1900's, the average person was getting 9 hours of sleep. Their sleep was more restful and free of the distractions and stressors of our current society. There was no TV, radio, internet, video games, cell phones, or other electronic gadgets to keep our brains on hyper-drive all the time. The people worked hard and then came home to read or play games with their family, preparing their brains for sleep. There was little shift work and the resultant disruption of our circadian rhythms. Their diet was healthier and free of additives and chemicals that hype up our brains. There was more daytime exercise and exposure to sunlight so that at night they were ready for sleep. Sleep disorders were a rare thing.

Move forward a century, and we have a totally different situation. The average person now is getting 6.5 hours of sleep. That is 2.5 hours less than a century ago. Is it any wonder we are exhausted? There are more patients with sleep disorders than we can count and we have a host of medical answers for them, including supplements, drugs, CPAP machines, biofeedback, relaxation classes, and psychotherapy. Where did all this poor sleep come from? We'll look at that later.

What does the Bible have to say about all of this? In Exodus 15:26, God tells the Jews coming out of Egyptian bondage after 400 years, *And He said, 'If you will give earnest heed to the voice of the Lord your God, and do what is right in His sight, and give ear to His commandments, and keep all His statutes, I will put none of the diseases on you which I have put on the Egyptians; for I, the Lord, am your healer.'* Could the Lord be telling America something? Have we listened to His voice lately? Have we done what is right in His sight? Have we obeyed His commandments? Have we kept all His statutes? I would argue a big "no" to all those questions. Well, He promised if we did these things we would not have the diseases (and the judgments) He put on the Egyptians to bring out His people. The contrary is also true. If we don't do these things, the Lord will allow us to get these diseases. He wants to be our Healer. Our nation must deserve it.

I still believe the Lord wants to heal His people despite our national disobedience. Christians are His people, adopted into His family as His sons and daughters. Jehovah-Rapha is just waiting for us to obey Him and ask for His healing. He has also given us knowledge of what we need to do to avoid and cure these diseases.

Can the government fix our health problems? There is no evidence that it has or can in the future. In fact, things are getting progressively worse, despite all the rhetoric. Throwing money at the problems is not helping; it never has and never will. There is a more fundamental issue. People have to want to change their lifestyle. That is an individual choice and can't be forced by the government. Yes, our government could be helping us by controlling all the food system and environmental toxins we are being exposed to. However, don't expect that any time soon

The Food and Drug Administration is supposed to be protecting us. The question is who are they protecting and from what? There is no evidence I can see that the FDA has done a good job at protecting Americans from toxic drugs, environmental poisons and food system toxins. In fact, under the FDA's watch, everything has gotten worse for our health. So, whom are they protecting? Follow the money trail. Big Pharmaceutical Companies? Big Agriculture? Big Chemical Companies? You decide.

I look at the government trying to fix our problems like a show at Sea World. I love to go to Sea World. I always make sure to go to the Sea Lion and Otter show. It is hysterical. There is always some kind of loose plot, but the animals are the stars. They are making noises, but no one can understand them. The people are trying to get them to do what they want, but sometimes it works and sometimes it does not. The animals do whatever they can to get the food they want. All the while the audience is laughing and being entertained and escaping from their problems for a little while. But when you leave the show, you are back to reality and the animals are back to their captivity…until the next show.

PFH Action Point

- **Thyroid and Autoimmune disorders are increasing at an alarming rate**
- **The majority of physician office visits are for anxiety and depression related complaints**
- **People complain that they are fatigued, have no energy, are in pain, and can't sleep well.**
- **Our government cannot fix these problems; you must take the steps needed to get healthy**

Chapter 3
IS THERE A CONSPIRACY?

My short answer is yes. However, the long answer may be different than you were thinking.

When we look at everything that has taken place since World War II in this country, and the subsequent decline in our health, there appears to be enough of a causal relationship that it begs the question: has there been a conspiracy to ruin our nation?

Let's look at some of the things that have happened since World War II:

- Our health has declined steadily and we are in the midst of an unprecedented health care crisis.
- There has been a progressive polluting and poisoning of our air, water, land and food.
- Drug and alcohol abuse are increasing to the point that most crime is somehow related and many of our ER visits are due to these.
- We have seen a decline in morality since the Bible and prayer were taken out of our schools and replaced with secular humanism and evolutionary theology. The result has been an explosion of sexually transmitted diseases and unwanted pregnancies.
- We have seen the devaluation of life resulting from legalized abortion and explicit violence in the media.

- The media is without restraint and explicit sex, violence, profanity and immorality appear on TV daily and our music is full of it; in fact, you can experience it any time by way of the internet.
- There has been a decline of the traditional family and it has been replaced with non-biblical concepts such as gay marriage
- Divorce is common and most homes are broken and children are being raised by a single mom; without a loving father, there is a high rate of crime and prison
- Violence and crime are escalating with criminals having access to military style weapons
- Government spending and our national debt are out of control and the US is a debtor nation
- We are engaged in wars we can't win and are dealing with the rise of Islamic terrorists that want to kill all Christians and Jews and destroy America. They are taught that if they do, or they die as a martyr in the process, Allah will bless them
- We have seen the decline of Biblical Christianity and the rise of a post-modern version that does not believe or follow what the Bible says

Let us use some sanctified imagination for a moment.

Imagine that Satan is having a meeting with his principalities right after World War II. He is not happy. Things did not turn out well.

In the beginning, things looked pretty good for the devil. His goal was not only world domination, but the extermination of every Jew and Christian. He wanted to destroy Christianity and everyone who worshipped the true God, Yhwh. You see, Satan hates the people of God and has been trying to destroy them for 2000 years. He had Hitler, who was a Satanist, working to kill every Jew and Christian he could and impose a godless religious system called Fascism. He had Japan working to ruthlessly conquer all of Asia and bring a false religion, Buddhism, to its peoples. It seemed like his plan was working and was unstoppable.

Enter the United States. It is clear that World War II would have turned out much differently if the US had not entered the war. In fact, if the US had not come to the aid of Europe, it would have fallen very soon. If we had not fought against Japanese tyranny, all of Asia would have fallen, as well. If the US had not rescued the Jews and Christians being slaughtered by Hitler, the Jewish people may have ceased to exist. Hitler was very close to developing an atomic bomb and had the rockets to carry them. If we had not entered the war when we did, things would have gotten very bad indeed.

It is clear that God rose up the United States for the purpose of defending the free world from Satan's agents. Not only were we founded as a Christian nation, we were also to be a haven for the Jewish people until they were able to come back to Palestine and form their own nation again. We have been the nation that has sent missionaries all over the world to spread the gospel of Jesus Christ. Our prosperity has resulted in enormous financial resources for ministries around the world helping those in need. We have printed and distributed more Bibles than can be counted. Our capacity to do good in the world has been unmatched in history.

Let's get back to our meeting. Satan is hot. The United States had ruined his plans again. World War I was not enough of a defeat, but now this. His principalities scramble for excuses.

"You guys are totally incompetent. I assign you this important task, and you blow it. I put you in charge of these nations and their leaders, empowering them with our spirit, so that those Christians and Jews would be eliminated forever. Instead, we lose everything!" said Satan.

"Boss, we are sorry. We did not anticipate the United States being able to affect our efforts like they did. We feel sure that if they had not had direct help from Him, they would have failed. No nation has ever done what they did to us," said the principality over Europe.

"Well, I am sick and tired of them ruining my agenda. They must be neutralized. I want a comprehensive plan to destroy the United States," said Satan.

"Boss, they are too strong now to make a military assault against them. We know we can get the communists in the Soviet Union and Asia to oppose them. But it is going to take more than that. They have a strong will to fight and win," said the principality over Russia.

"Yes. It is going to take a multifaceted approach to take them down. Perhaps no attack from the outside will destroy them. I think their destruction needs to come from within," said Satan.

"How about we corrupt their government with greedy politicians and agencies that don't protect the people and cut back on their military?" asked the principality over South America.

"That is good, but we have tried that before. We need more. Something we have not done before. Something that will take away their will and leave them vulnerable," said Satan.

"How about we get them all so sick that they have no health or energy to serve the churches they go to? Perhaps they will even stop going. They will stop volunteering and going on mission trips. We can get their pastors and spouses sick so that they have to drop out of ministry or stop many of their activities. Everyone will get fat and fatigued and so obsessed with their chronic illnesses that they don't have the time or energy to help others. Everyone will get anxious and depressed and be put on medications instead of dealing with their issues. Their nation will fall apart from within," said the principality from North America.

"I like it," said Satan. "We can even ruin their healthcare system so that the people don't really ever get better, but just take a lot of medicines with side effects that further ruin their health. There will be no emphasis on preventive care, just symptom management"

"We can have the government make decisions that protect chemical companies, pharmaceutical companies, and agricultural companies so that they can poison the environment, the food supply, and the water," said the principality over Africa.

"Yes. Let's think this through. What if we also get prayer and the Bible thrown out of their schools? We'll replace it with evolution and other godless myths and brainwash their kids. Think of it. Their morals will decline, abortions will increase, life will be devalued, sexual diseases will run rampant, families will fall apart and divorces will be common. People will turn to drugs and alcohol to deal with their hurts and turn away from religion. Then, they will get even sicker!" said Satan.

"With that, violent crimes will increase and their prisons will be filled. We can ruin even more lives," said the principality over the South Pacific.

"I suggest the rise of Islam and terrorism so that the country will be in fear of attacks from radicals and withdraw from the world scene as its protector. Israel will be under constant threats, with its principal ally impotent, until its neighbors destroy it. We will engage the US in wars that they can't win until we break the will of their sickened people," said the principality over the Middle East.

"I also suggest infiltrating their seminaries with our demons to inject a liberal, non-biblical theology that will poison generations of their pastors and ultimately ruin their evangelical churches. They will think everything is going well for them while they are really on a path straight to hell! They will reject the authority of the Bible as we raise all kinds of stupid objections to it. They will adopt laws and appoint leaders who will give them what they want. We can secularize their nation and create a post-modern, humanistic society with no morals. We can do that in Europe, too," said the principality over Europe.

"Remember what we did to bring down Rome? We can do the same things again since the US and Rome are so similar. We got them rich and fat and comfortable. We got them obsessed with sports and the games and their stars. We encouraged them to live out all kinds of immoral lifestyles with the approval of the government. We taxed the middle class to death and everyone became dependent on the government without any incentive to work. We created a volunteer army that only the worst people would join and had no heart to fight with it. When our hordes of barbarians came, they had no will to fight. We can do the same things here," said Satan.

"We can get them distracted and obsessed with technology and the media and poison them with our ideas. We'll get them hooked on aliens and vampires. We'll have their celebrities push New Age philosophies and false religions that we will create. Imagine what would happen if we hammer them with sex, violence, immorality, greed, and profanity. It would be beautiful," said the principality over Russia.

"I like all of your ideas," said Satan. "We need to do all of it. Start immediately. It will take a few decades for us to start seeing the fruit, but I envision a time when the United States will become impotent. Then, we can unleash a war like the world has never seen and they will be unable to ruin our plans again. Death to the Jews. Death to the Christians. I will be in control of this world and all the people will follow me and we will defeat Jesus at Armageddon. I will be God!"

While this sounds like fiction, I am not so sure. When you look at the decisions that have been made in this nation and the condition we are in, there seems to have been a master plan to ruin us. Yes, there are secret societies behind the scenes that are manipulating things. But they are tools of the devil. He has created the master plan.

What can we do? We must fight back. We can start by taking control of our health and making the right decisions to get us healthy. Yes, there are things that need to be done to fix our government, the environment, healthcare, the debt, the church and its liberal teachings, immorality, the media, foreign policy and many other things. Most of us are not in a position to fix those. However, we can affect the health of our families by learning more and making the right choices.

Chapter 4
THE BOTTOM LINE

In previous chapters we have been examining the state of our health here in America and the problems that we are facing as individuals and as a nation. It is clear that we are facing enormous challenges that require us to take a radically different look at how we approach healthcare and our health.

I invite you into the world of Functional Medicine. This is a relatively new term that I don't expect most of you to be familiar with. It is not Alternative Medicine, which is the rejection of western medical philosophy and the science it was founded on, and replacing it with alternative treatments that have little scientific basis. While these alternative medicine treatments may provide some help to select patients on a temporary basis, they are rooted in philosophies and religious practices that are the antithesis to my Christian beliefs.

Functional Medicine, or Complementary Medicine, is the integration of traditional western medical diagnosis and treatment with natural therapies that heal. Functional Medicine seeks to get to the root cause or the very bottom of what I call the Diagnosis Inverted Pyramid. I envision most patients in America are being treated in a healthcare system that emphasizes symptom management. So, if the symptoms are all at the top of the Diagnosis Inverted Pyramid, then our goal should be to search for their causes. As you do that, you eventually get to the apex of the Diagnosis Inverted Pyramid, which is the bottom line.

Diagnosis Inverted Pyramid

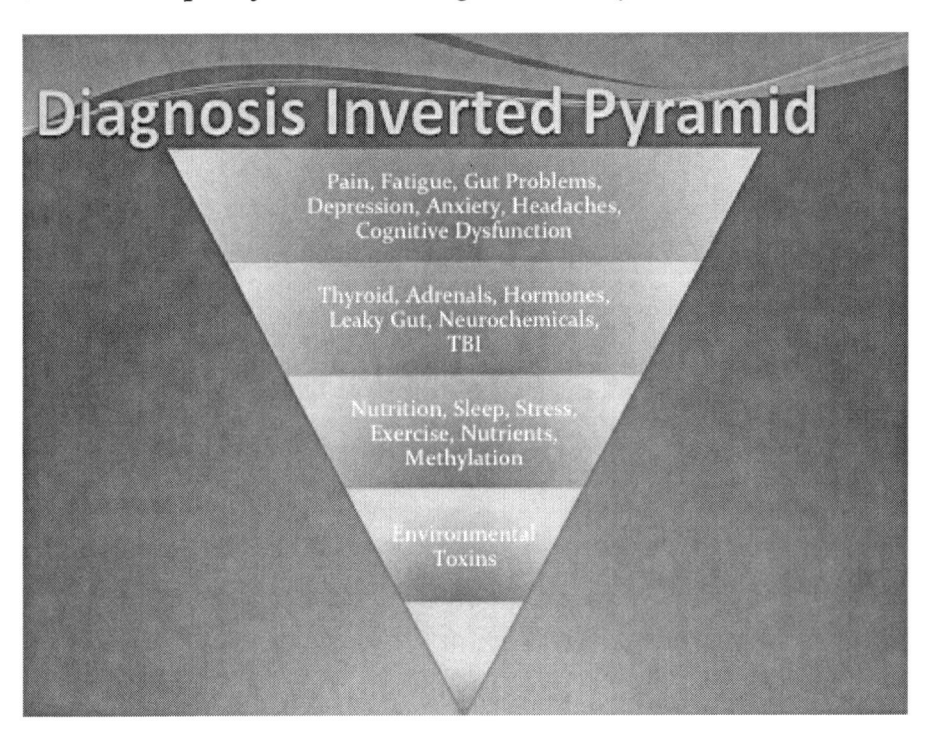

- Pain, Fatigue, Gut Problems, Depression, Anxiety, Headaches, Cognitive Dysfunction
- Thyroid, Adrenals, Hormones, Leaky Gut, Neurochemicals, TBI
- Nutrition, Sleep, Stress, Exercise, Nutrients, Methylation
- Environmental Toxins

Let's look at an example. A patient presents to a typical primary care office with a complaint of pain all over and fatigue. During the interview, it is discovered that the patient also has headaches, abdominal pain, and constipation. They are depressed, anxious, and mental fog. These are the symptoms that would occupy the top of the Diagnosis Inverted Pyramid. Several diagnostic tests are ordered on the patient in a cursory attempt to rule out treatable causes for the condition. Typically these screening laboratory tests will come back normal and the patient will be diagnosed with Fibromyalgia. Then begins the symptom management with numerous prescription medications, including perhaps opioid (narcotic) pain medications.

In Functional Medicine, we seek to find the causes of the condition rather than just manage the symptoms. So, for this case, the next step would be a more thorough investigation to seek the underlying causes. Typically, the next layer down in the Diagnosis Inverted Pyramid would be conditions such as thyroid, adrenal and hormone imbalances. Other problems would include Leaky Gut, Neurochemical imbalances, or a history of a Traumatic Brain Injury (TBI). Going further down, we will find that those would be caused by poor nutritional choices, sleep dysfunction, stress, lack of exercise, nutrient deficiencies and Methylation disorders. The apex of the Diagnosis Inverted Pyramid usually turns out to be environmental toxins. These will include Biotoxins, Persistent Organic Pollutants (POP's), Endocrine Disruptors, heavy metals, and food chain toxins. In this model, once you correct the underlying causes at the bottom, the symptoms at the top improve.

Functional Medicine is like being a medical detective. There has to be an exhaustive search for clues and the accumulation of evidence to discover who committed the crime. In this case, we need to discover how the patient got sick and what needs to be done to correct the problems. Using a Functional Medicine approach, it is clear to me that the underlying cause of most of our chronic health problems in this country is **inflammation**. If we can defeat **inflammation**, we can defeat most of the chronic diseases that are robbing our people of their vitality and quality of life. They are also the diseases that are responsible for most of our healthcare expenditures and are costing business and industry untold billions of dollars in lost productivity.

Again, using our Functional Medicine paradigm, let us put on our medical detective hat and find the underlying causes of this **inflammation**. I want to tell you about five specific culprits: Free Radicals, nutrient deficiencies, food chain toxins, environmental toxins, and Biotoxins. Let's take a look at each of these in detail. By addressing these culprits and correcting them, the underlying **inflammation** will resolve and so will most of our health issues.

PFH Action Point

- **Functional Medicine seeks to treat the cause of the condition, rather than the symptoms**
- **I utilize the Diagnosis Inverted Pyramid to trace the condition back to the cause**

- The underlying cause of most of our chronic health problems is inflammation
- The causes of inflammation include Free Radicals, nutrient deficiencies, food chain toxins, environmental toxins, and Biotoxins
- By addressing these causes, our inflammation and chronic conditions will resolve

1. Free Radicals

Most of you have probably heard about Free Radicals at some point in the last few years, however you may not totally understand what they are and their role in **inflammation**. Free Radicals are chemically active atoms or molecular fragments. They have a charge due to an excess or deficient number of electrons. They are very unstable and scavenge the body to get or donate electrons. In the process of scavenging the body, they cause damage to cells, proteins, and your DNA. Another term for this is oxidative damage. Oxidative damage is the same process that causes iron to rust, or an apple to turn brown, when they are exposed to the air.

Where do these Free Radicals come from? Some Free Radicals are produced within our own bodies. We call this endogenous production. Free Radicals are produced from aerobic respiration, metabolism, infection, and strenuous exercise. Free Radicals can also be created from **inflammation**, so that the process is self-perpetuating.

Free Radicals are also produced from our exposure to outside sources, what we call exogenous sources. These include Endocrine Disruptors. Some Endocrine Disruptors are Persistent Organic Pollutants (POP's) such as plastics, solvents and pesticides. Heavy metals, such as mercury, lead, and arsenic are other culprits. Exposure to chemical pollution of the air, ground, and water creates Free Radicals. Ultraviolet radiation, such as from sunlight, x-rays and radiation therapy, and iodizing radiation all produce Free Radicals. Exposure to smoking, alcohol and drugs, as well as the contaminants in them, will produce Free Radicals. Finally, food additives and preservatives contribute to Free Radical production.

Free Radicals are constantly attacking our cells and our DNA. Some tissues of our body, such as the lining of our intestinal tract, may be exposed to Free Radical attack 100,000 times per day. Under this constant assault, it is amazing that any of our cells survive.

Once a Free Radical enters the human body, it can combine with oxygen to form a Reactive Oxygen Species. These are the most biologically active and damaging Free Radicals. They include hydrogen peroxide, hypochlorous acid, singlet oxygen, superoxide, and the hydroxyl radical.

God, in all of His wisdom, created for us a defense system against these Free Radicals. Our defense involves substances called antioxidants. Antioxidants neutralize one or more of these Reactive Oxygen Species. Some antioxidants are produced within our own bodies, such as Glutathione. However, most antioxidants must be consumed in our foods. The more antioxidants we have on board, the more Free Radicals will be neutralized and the less damage to our cells and DNA. In order to stop the **inflammation** caused by Free Radicals, we must have adequate antioxidants.

PFH Action Point

- **Free Radicals attack our cells and DNA and cause oxidative damage**
- **While we make some Free Radicals, most come from external sources**
- **POP's, heavy metals, Pollution, UV Radiation, food additives, alcohol and smoking are major sources**
- **Antioxidants neutralize Free Radicals and we must consume a lot of them**

2. Nutrient Deficiencies

A second cause of **inflammation** is nutrient deficiencies. People in the United States consume a diet that we have been told is very healthy and full of nutrients. Many countries envy our abundance of food and the fact that we can go down the street to a store and buy anything we want. I do most of the food shopping in my home and I actually enjoy going to the supermarket to purchase healthy foods for my family. However, as you look around the store, it becomes obvious that most of the foods there are nutrient deficient. How can this be?

The vast majority of the produce grown in the United States is grown in nutrient depleted soil. We have just not done a good enough job of replacing essential nutrients in the soil. There has been no time for the soil to rest and be replenished. Crop after crop is planted and harvested without any regard for the nutrient content of the food produced. In ancient Israel, God commanded the people to farm the land for six years and then take one year to rest the land. It was this failure to rest the land in the Old Testament that partially resulted in God's prophecy to Daniel of the "70 weeks" of punishment for Israel.

Two nutrient deficiencies that have occurred, due to failure to replenish these nutrients in our soil, are iodine and selenium. It used to be that iodine deficiency in the United States was confined to an area called the "Goiter belt" which was located around the Great Lakes in the Midwest. There was no natural iodine in the soil there; thus, there was widespread iodine deficiency resulting in thyroid disease and goiters. I have had several older patients tell me of growing up in that area and the great prevalence of goiters and thyroid disease. In fact, they recall sitting in school classrooms and the teachers handing out iodine tablets to all of the students daily.

Once the United States began a program to put iodine in our salt, things got a little better. The goiters became less common, but the thyroid disease did not. You just don't obtain very much iodine in the salt that you consume. In fact, because of the low salt craze that has swept through our nation, people are not getting enough iodine. Because of over farming, all of the soil in the United States is now iodine deficient. This is a major cause of the epidemic thyroid disease in this nation that we discussed earlier.

Another nutrient that has been depleted from the soil is Selenium. Many of you have not probably heard much about Selenium, but it is an extremely critical nutrient. Selenium is an important part of our immune system. It also has an important role to play in detoxification, mostly in our liver. Selenium is critical for the proper functioning of iodine in your thyroid gland. Unfortunately, because of the Selenium deficiency of our soil, many of us are all Selenium deficient.

Another cause of nutrient deficiencies is the picking of our produce in an unripe state. While this helps with the long transportation and storage issues of getting produce to the market, it has not allowed the fruits and vegetables to ripen naturally and produce the optimum amount of nutrients. I don't know about you, but I hate going to the store and seeing a table of unripe produce and having to pick through it to find something that is not green. In order to fool us into thinking that the produce is ripe, the food industry will typically use carbon dioxide or other gases to try to ripen them artificially on their way to the store. In addition, long transportation and storage times further depress nutrient levels in our fruits and vegetables.

Another source of nutrient deficiencies is the consumption of fast food, canned and processed foods. The heating, cooking, frying, and processing of foods will greatly lower nutrient levels, especially for very sensitive heat unstable nutrients. This is a major source of the health problems in our nation. Americans are obsessed with fast food and highly processed foods. While they are convenient, and take less time than preparing a meal of fresh produce, they are devoid of many nutrients that are essential for our bodies to function properly.

There are numerous toxins that we are exposed to that bind essential nutrients. This binding can occur both in our foods and in our bodies. The list includes many plastics and heavy metals. We will be taking a look at these toxins shortly.

Another problem that is occurring more frequently in the United States is Leaky Gut Syndrome. This has been called various names in the past including Irritable Bowel Syndrome, Functional Bowel Syndrome and Spastic Colon. Leaky Gut Syndrome involves the **inflammation** of our intestinal lining resulting in poor absorption of nutrients. Common symptoms include pain, spasm, bloating, diarrhea, and constipation. Because of Leaky Gut Syndrome, I commonly see nutrient deficiencies including iron, magnesium, calcium, and various vitamins.

In our attempt to compensate for these nutrient deficiencies, we often resort to various supplements, including multivitamins. We will be taking a closer look at supplements later. For now, just know that not all supplements are created equal. In fact it is well documented that many solid tablet supplements pass through your intestinal tract totally intact and never get absorbed. Because of Leaky Gut Syndrome, supplements may also not be readily absorbed. Thus, the nutrient deficiencies continue.

PFH Action Point

- **Nutrient deficiencies are rampant in our country**
- **Iodine, Selenium, and other essential nutrients have been farmed out of the soil**
- **How we farm, pick and transport food affects their nutrient levels**
- **Fast food, processed food, and toxins deplete nutrient levels**
- **Leaky Gut and other malabsorption disorders cause deficiencies in nutrients**

3. Food Chain Toxins

Our food chain has been contaminated. Unless you are growing your own organic produce, you are in danger of exposure to toxins in our food chain at every meal. Let us take a look at some of these toxins.

Pesticides are big business. Millions of gallons of toxic pesticides are sprayed on our crops in the United States every year. Even more concerning are the pesticides that are sprayed on crops that we import from other countries. Unless you are eating organic produce from a reliable source, you are consuming pesticides. We will be examining what those pesticides do to your body later as we examine the subject of Endocrine Disruptors. For now, just remember that most of these pesticides were originally developed as nerve gas agents to be used in warfare and are deadly, not only to insects and other pests, but also to human beings.

The subject of Genetically Modified Organisms (GMOs) is complicated. We will also be looking at this in more detail later. My feeling is that we are living in a big lab experiment with companies producing genetically modified foods and releasing them into the food chain to see what will happen to us. There has not been any substantial testing for safety. Could it be that the explosion of food allergies, Leaky Gut Syndrome, Autism, ADHD, and other health issues are related to the release of GMO foods into our food chain?

The introduction of hormones into the food chain has greatly altered the health of our people. In an attempt to increase profits by growing our meats faster and with more bulk, the food industry has ruined the hormone systems of countless women and men in the United States. Most of the hormones introduced are either Growth Hormone or Estrogen derivatives.

This is one of the causes for the increase in Estrogen Dominance among women in the United States, especially young girls. Do you ever wonder why our daughters are having their menstrual periods very early and growing breasts at very young ages? This is the major reason. All those years that we were feeding our families chicken because we thought it was better for them than beef. Who would have ever thought that the hormones in the chicken were affecting the health of our families? While it is becoming easier to buy hormone free meats and dairy products than it was several years ago, it is still more costly. You also have very little control of what you eat when you go out to a restaurant. Unless they advertise that they are using products free of hormones, you can be sure that they are not.

The introduction of antibiotics into the food chain has altered the health of this country forever. The routine use of antibiotics in our animals has resulted in the emergence of superbugs that are resistant to antibiotics. This has caused us huge headaches in our hospitals. Patients are dying because the antibiotics no longer work on the organisms they are infected with. While it is getting easier to purchase meats and dairy products that are free of antibiotics, it is more expensive. Why hasn't the government taken action to stop the routine use of antibiotics and hormones in our food chain?

Bacterial contamination of our food chain is widespread. Whether it is at the place of harvest, the food processing plant, the supermarket, or at the restaurant, bacterial contamination can occur fairly easily. We have all heard the media reports of recalls of vast amounts of meat and produce. This not only is a tremendous waste of resources, given the amount of hungry people in the world, but an enormous financial loss. Many people suffer needlessly from illnesses due to the contamination of their food with bacteria. While we should be aware of proper cleansing and storage of our foods in our homes, we can't control what happens before the food reaches us.

PFH Action Point

- **Food chain toxins are everywhere**
- **Pesticides are Endocrine Disruptors and are on our produce**
- **GMO foods have been introduced into the food chain with no data they are safe**
- **Hormones are wrecking our Endocrine systems and causing cancer**
- **Antibiotics have created a nightmare of drug resistant organisms**
- **Bacterial contamination is common, resulting in illness and financial loss**

Food additives are big business. Stabilizing agents, colors, flavors, and other chemicals are packed into our foods, especially highly processed foods. Just what are these things and how do they impact our health? Environmental Working Group recently did a nice review of some of these chemicals and called it the *Dirty Dozen Guide to Food Additives*. It is available on their website. You will be shocked. Let's take a look at a few things commonly found on ingredient lists.

Nitrates and Nitrites are commonly found in processed foods as coloring agents, preservatives and flavoring. They are particularly obvious in cured meats like salami, ham, bacon, sausage, and hot dogs. They can react with proteins in the food or in your body and form nitrosamines, which cause cancer. The World Health Organization (WHO) declared these agents as probable human carcinogens. They need to be avoided entirely.

Many of my patients have reactions to Nitrates and Nitrites as well as another common preservative, Sulfites. I can tell you that if I am exposed to Sulfites in particular, I will break out in hives. For many people, it is dose dependent. This means that the more you consume, the more reaction you will have. You may not have a reaction at very low levels. Many processed foods contain Sulfites; particularly be wary of wines. These agents become Free Radicals and directly damage our cells, causing cancer.

Potassium Bromate is added to dough to strengthen it and help it rise during baking. California lists it as a known carcinogen and it is not allowed in food in Canada, the United Kingdom, and the European Union. Why does the FDA still allow this in our flour? Bromine is also a thyroid goitrogen (toxin) and interferes with the production of thyroid hormone. We will be looking at that later. This must be avoided.

How does an Endocrine Disruptor like Propyl Paraben get into our food supply? A federal study found 91% of Americans had detectable amounts in their urine. It has been found in half of the foods in our stores. The FDA classifies it as "Generally Recognized as Safe" or GRAS for short. How did that happen when it acts as a weak estrogen, interfering with hormone function, and accelerating cancer cell growth?

There is a problem with the FDA's approval system for GRAS additives. You need to avoid it.

Butylated hydroxyanisole (BHA) and Butylated hydroxytoluene (BHT) are commonly found on ingredient lists, especially chips, preserved meats and foods containing fats. They are touted as preservatives, but there is nothing preserving about what they do to us. BHA is recognized as a potential carcinogen by many organizations and the EU considers it an Endocrine Disruptor, affecting hormone and thyroid function. BHT also has evidence that it may be a carcinogen and has similar Endocrine Disruptor effects on hormone and thyroid function. They can also affect behavior. Propyl gallate is a preservative used in edible fat products, such as sausage and lard. There is evidence it causes tumors and is an Endocrine Disruptor. All of these should be avoided.

Theobromine is an alkaloid commonly found in commercial, processed chocolate that has effects similar to caffeine. It was given a GRAS designation without FDA approval through a loophole. People consume a lot of this and the health effects are really unknown. We will discuss later about the difference between healthy and unhealthy chocolate. For now, know that most chocolate you buy in the stores is very unhealthy and contains fats, sugar and additives that are harming your health.

What are "natural flavors" and "artificial flavors"? You will find these terms listed on most processed food ingredient lists. Have you ever wondered what they are? Well, there is no way to know, as the manufacturer does not typically divulge that information. Besides whatever ingredients they are using as flavors, there are "incidental additives" like emulsifiers, solvents (like propylene glycol), and preservatives (like BHA and BHT). All told, there could be up to 100 distinct substances in these flavoring mixtures. Who knows what effects these substances are having on the health of your family. What about food allergies to these undisclosed substances? Avoid products having these "natural" and "artificial" flavors listed.

The Bottom Line

Citric acid appears on many ingredient lists. It sounds good, right? It sounds like it comes from citrus fruits and is naturally derived, doesn't it? Nothing could be further from the truth. Let me describe to you for a few minutes how citric acid is made. By the way, citric acid may be called ascorbic acid, or vitamin C, and could be in your vitamins. It is also used as a flavoring agent, giving things a more crisp or tart flavor, and as a preservative.

Aspergillus niger, a naturally occurring black mold, has been genetically modified and exposed to gamma radiation in order to make strains that produce more citric acid. Thus, citric acid is a mycotoxin, or a toxin produced by mold. We will look at that later. It is placed on a medium of GMO corn, which is often exposed to a mercury-containing alkali. The three most common mercury-contaminated food ingredients are high fructose corn syrup (HFCS), sodium benzoate and citric acid. We'll look at HFCS in detail later. Remember this contamination with mercury the next time you read an ingredient list that mentions these agents.

To purify the corn syrup, acids and heat are often employed, including the use of an iron/cyanide compound. That's right, cyanide can be used to make citric acid. The Aspergillus niger is applied to ferment the corn syrup over several days and produce the citric acid. The culture broth is then separated and calcium hydroxide applied to precipitate calcium citrate. Sulfuric acid is then applied to produce the citric acid. A process of crystallization makes it ready for market to be used in a host of products. A by-product of this process can be sodium citrate, which you will also see on ingredient lists, formed by applying sodium hydroxide (lye) to the citric acid.

One of the by-products of the use of citric acid in sodas, sport drinks and citrus-flavored beverages is benzene. This is a human carcinogen, causing all kinds of health problems, and occurs as a result of the interaction of citric acid with sodium or potassium benzoate, another common ingredient. It occurs right in the container. Do not drink anything that contains these two ingredients together. Actually, you should not drink anything that has any of the ingredients we have just discussed.

Another flavoring agent is MSG, or monosodium glutamate. While we have known for many years that some people react in a violent way to MSG, particularly with allergic reactions, I believe the problem is much more widespread than that. I believe that there are many lower grade reactions to MSG with unusual symptoms that are not the typical allergic reaction. The backlash against MSG became so great that the food industry found ways to call it something different. The current ideology is to include it in "natural flavoring" on the food label. MSG is particularly a problem with oriental food restaurants and any type of packaged oriental foods. If the restaurant you are dining at will not make your meal without MSG, you need to find a new restaurant. Beware that in many Chinese restaurants, the egg rolls and soups are already premade with MSG and it cannot be removed. MSG can have profound effects on brain function and behavior.

Diacetyl is a flavoring agent used particularly as a butter flavor in microwave popcorn. It is also used in yogurt, cheese, butterscotch, maple, and fruit flavorings like strawberry and raspberry. Workers exposed to Diacetyl are developing lung disease in large numbers. If it is doing that to the workers from breathing it, what is it doing to those of us who ingest it? Beware of butter flavors and other non-specific "flavor" ingredients. Harmful chemicals often lurk behind the term.

Regarding artificial sweeteners, I can tell you unequivocally that they are toxins in our food chain. While we will be examining these in more detail later, Aspartame, Saccharin, and Sucralose need to be avoided entirely.

Many of you have probably heard the controversy regarding food colors, known as FD&C colors. These include, red, yellow, caramel and others. These synthetic chemical colors are used to make food look more appealing and vibrant. They may be listed under the term "artificial color." Many have believed for years that red dyes were responsible for abnormal behavior in children. I believe this is true about many of these coloring agents. It is amazing when you take hyperactive children off of sugar and food colors, how much better they get. Something that is made in the laboratory to color your food cannot be very good for you. These artificial food colors often times appear on the ingredient list of processed foods, including so called "natural foods". If the foods are so natural, why do they need an artificial color to make them more appealing? There are associations between these colors, and the contaminants in them, and cancer. Try to eliminate them from your diet.

Other additives include phosphates and aluminum. Phosphates are widely used in processed foods and fast foods and high phosphate consumption is linked to heart disease. It is definitely a problem for those with kidney disease. Sodium aluminum phosphate, sodium aluminum sulfate, and other aluminum derivatives are used as food stabilizers. High levels of aluminum cause behavioral and neurologic problems. There appears to be a link to the development of Alzheimer's dementia and other neurodegenerative disorders. Phosphate and aluminum additives are best avoided.

PFH Action Point

- **Food additives and preservatives in processed and fast foods are hurting us and must be avoided**
- **Many of these additives cause cancer, are Endocrine Disruptors, and cause neurologic and behavioral problems**
- **Some food additives can cause life threatening allergic reactions**
- **We must be diligent to eliminate these toxins by eating less processed foods and reading ingredient lists**

Let's look at some examples of how foods and food chain toxins cause **inflammation**. A high carbohydrate meal induces an immediate increase in Free Radicals, endothelial dysfunction (blood vessel spasm and damage), and sympathetic hyperactivity. A diet high in omega 6 fatty acids, and low in omega 3 fatty acids, will produce pro-inflammatory eicosanoids and cytokines and reduce anti-inflammatory mediators. Consuming trans fatty acids increases triglycerides and LDL cholesterol, pro-inflammatory cytokines, and insulin resistance.

How about nutrient deficiencies? Low Magnesium intake and poor absorption results in reduced ATP (energy production), increased Free Radical, increased pro-inflammatory eicosanoids and cytokines, and increased pain. Low Potassium intake results in low oxygen levels, increased Free Radical production, tissue acidity, and insulin resistance. Low Phytonutrient intake (antioxidants), by not consuming them in our diet, results in increased Free Radicals from an inability to neutralize them; the result is **inflammation**. Lack of good gut bacteria (Probiotics), from poor diet, antibiotic and toxin exposure results in the overgrowth of Candida (yeast) and bad bacteria; the result is endotoxemia and systemic **inflammation**. Low serum vitamin D3 levels results in decreased anti-inflammatory cytokines, increased pro-inflammatory cytokines, and pain.

As we can see, our diet greatly impacts the level of **inflammation** in our bodies. Since **inflammation** is the ultimate cause of pain, diet also impacts our pain levels. By the same reasoning, an Anti-inflammatory diet and lifestyle will reduce **inflammation** and pain. We will be examining each of these in detail later.

PFH Action Point

- **Foods and food chain toxins, like a high carbohydrate diet, high omega 6 fatty acid intake, and consuming trans fatty acids, increase inflammation**
- **Nutrient deficiencies, like low Magnesium, low Potassium, and low antioxidants increase inflammation**
- **Lack of Probiotic bacteria increases inflammation**
- **Low serum vitamin D3 levels increase inflammation**

Chapter 5
Our Toxic World

In our last chapter, I discussed with you how **inflammation** is the apex of our diagnosis inverted pyramid and the cause of most of the chronic diseases in this country. We looked at the five causes of **inflammation**. The first three were Free Radicals, nutrient deficiencies, and food chain toxins. The last two are so important and immense that I thought that they deserved a separate chapter.

We live in a chemical soup. As I have studied what we have done to our environment, and the mess that we are living in, that was the only conclusion that I could come to. The amount of toxins that we are exposed to on a daily basis is staggering. These toxic exposures greatly affect our health and the health of our families. They are not something that can just be ignored and believe that they will just go away and not affect us. Our chemical soup is getting worse by the day.

Occasionally I enjoy cooking. One of the things that I like to do is to make a big pot of soup. Now this is not just any soup. I put a lot of thought into what goes in this. Basically, I take whatever leftovers I have in the freezer that need to be used and start from that point. Oftentimes this is some organic turkey that I made and have not quite gotten to yet. Sometimes I will use ground organic bison as the base. What happens next is unpredictable. I get as many vegetables as I can find and put them in, dicing and chopping for hours. Again these may be things that have been in the freezer for a while and need to be used. When I am done, I have a very thick soup that more resembles a stew.

When I think about the condition of our environment and what we are living in, I can easily draw an analogy to my special soup. It seems like chemical companies, pharmaceutical companies, and big agricultural companies have thrown in every toxic and harmful chemical and food that they have into a big pot and created a toxic soup. Without telling us, they have made us an ingredient in the soup. One of the things that I discovered in making my soup, is that the longer it simmers the more the flavors blend together. Then you add some spices and you have your final product. If the soup is made correctly it can be very healthy. In the case of our toxic soup, the flavors have all blended together to create something that is very unhealthy.

In order to understand the concepts of toxicity, we first need to go over a few definitions. My goal is not to make you environmental medicine specialists, but we need to have some basic understanding of genetics.

Let's start with the term Epigenomics. While this sounds like a very complicated subject, it basically comes down to how environment shapes our structure and function. God has created us with a wonderful blueprint for life called DNA. Our DNA is broken up into smaller segments called genes. These genes code for the production of specific proteins and enzymes that affect the structure and function of our body down to the tiniest detail. The human genome is the sum total of these genes. What we have learned over time is that our genes have been encoded by our Creator to make us a certain way. However, our environment can alter the expression of these genes.

What we are describing here is really called adaptation, which is the way an organism adapts to its environment. Thus, our environment affects how our genes are expressed. So how we turn out is a function of both our DNA and the environment we live in. We are not talking about natural selection. Natural selection is a concept from evolutionary theory. I remember when I was a brainwashed proponent of evolution. Now, I can look back and realize how badly I had been deceived. There is no evidence that evolution takes place.

No species has ever changed into another species, which is the major tenant that evolution hangs on. Evolution teaches that random chance mutations, over long periods of time, result in changes in structure and function that increase the competitive advantage of an animal or plant. The survival of the fittest assures that these beneficial mutations will be passed on to their offspring. A species eventually changes into another species and that is how we came about. Humans are descended from pond scum, fish, reptiles, and monkeys. What is the evidence? The evidence is that animals and plants do adapt to their environment, but they do not change into another species.

It is hard to believe that at one time in my life I was a devout atheist. I believed in evolution and that there was no God, only cosmic accidents leading to the creation of life. The problem was that there was absolutely no evidence that what I was taught, and what I believed, were true. It sounded good for someone not wanting to believe in God, because I would then have to live by His rules. It was far better just not to believe God existed and that I was just descended from animals and could live the way I wanted. I wanted to be able to make my own rules.

When I finally began to look at the hard evidence that evolution was a bad theory with no scientific or experiential support, I had to overcome a lot of bias and bad personal moral and lifestyle choices. But, the facts are the facts. There is no fossil evidence (despite the discovery of millions of fossils) that any species has ever changed into another species. There is no missing link. There is also no evidence that we are becoming more developed over time. Instead, as the Second Law of Thermodynamics indicates, things are decaying and becoming less complex, a process called entropy. If God were not intervening in our universe, everything would deteriorate and cease to exist.

The current term used to describe our belief in special creation and a Creator is Intelligent Design. There are a lot of really good scientists and smart people behind this. I don't put myself in that elite category, but as a physician I do have some degree of intelligence and have gathered many experiences in the real world. Intelligent Design just makes sense. Evolution does not.

When we look at DNA, for example, it is apparent that it could not have just evolved over millions of years, as I was taught. Here are microscopic strands of the most complex codes in the universe inhabiting every cell in our bodies. By way of only four amino acids in different sequences, God has encoded every cell with the information needed to make an entire person, down to the most infinitely small detail. There are systems to turn off and on the genes on the DNA as needed by our bodies so that only a portion is used at a time. There are repair and protection mechanisms to prevent mutations, since most of them are bad. Yet evolutionists would have us believe that mutations are good and have resulted in our DNA progressively getting more advanced, eventually resulting in people. The evidence does not agree.

Let's go back to adaptation. As our environment has been progressively poisoned, our bodies have tried to adapt to these changes. However, the toxins are more numerous and destructive than our bodies can handle. God created us with many complex mechanisms to detoxify bad things that get into our bodies. The problem is that many of the toxins we are dealing with today do not have natural detoxification mechanisms because they are man-made toxins. These toxins have caused changes in how our genome (DNA) is expressed. The study of how toxins have affected our genome to cause acute and chronic diseases is called Toxigenomics.

As we learn more about how cancer cells develop and reproduce to form tumors and eventually kill us, it becomes clear that toxins play a major role in these processes. Since 1 in 3 Americans will receive a diagnosis of cancer in their lifetimes, it is critically important that we understand how to prevent this from happening. While diet, lifestyle, genetics, and some viruses clearly contribute to the development of cancer, exposure to toxins has been misunderstood and under-emphasized. The process of a cell changing from a normal cell to a cancer cell is called carcinogenesis.

The Halifax Project has caused us to rethink how carcinogens affect our cells and ultimately result in cancer. This was an effort to bring together over 300 researchers from 31 countries to look at new approaches to cancer therapy and low dose exposures to common chemicals and their role in cancer development. They identified ten distinct steps, called the Hallmarks of Cancer, involved in the change of a cell from a normal one to a precancerous cell to a cancerous cell. Along the way there are genetic mutations and other genetic changes to the cell.

Thus, the development of cancer is a multi-step process that does not occur all at once, but over many years. There are multiple "hits" to the cell resulting in changes and progression in each Hallmark of Cancer step. The last step is **inflammation**, which is the subject of this book. Chronic **inflammation** can result in the right environment for cancer cell survival, proliferation (spreading), and angiogenesis (production of new blood vessels to supply the tumor). **Inflammation** also results in Free Radical production, which further damages DNA.

The results of the Halifax Project raise very disturbing issues. They looked at 85 chemicals that are known to trigger cancer-related hallmark processes. While we know that certain chemicals and heavy metals can cause cancer by themselves due to sufficient exposure over a certain period of time, it is more disturbing that so-called "probably safe" chemicals and low levels of exposure can cause cancer by working together on different parts of the cell's cancer-related hallmark processes. They found that 59% of these 85 chemicals do affect cancer hallmark processes at low doses. Thus, low dose combinations of chemical toxins may be more important than a high dose exposure to just one bad toxin.

Environmental Working Group has published an excellent summary of the Halifax Project findings and a Dirty Dozen list of harmful chemicals for us to avoid to prevent cancer. They found that 23 of the 85 chemicals studied by the Halifax Project are currently being detected in the bodies of sample patients around the US by the Centers for Disease Control and Prevention (CDC). The Dirty Dozen list includes BPA, atrazine, organophosphate pesticides, phthalates, lead, mercury, PFC's, PBDE's, triclosan and nonylphenol. We will be examining each of them.

There are several major areas of environmental toxins I want to tell you about as they directly affect your health and the health of your families. Remember, the effects of exposures, even at low levels, are additive over time. So it is very important to eliminate as many of these toxins as you can to prevent cancer and other diseases.

PFH Action Point

- **We live in a chemical soup**
- **These toxins affect our DNA (genome), causing damage and changes in how it is expressed**
- **The Halifax Project has caused us to rethink how cancer cells develop**
- **Multiple toxic hits over time cause changes to the cells that result in their becoming cancer cells; it is not just usually one exposure**
- **You must reduce your exposure to all toxins to prevent cancer**

4. Endocrine Disruptors

Let us first take a look at Endocrine Disruptors. Endocrine Disruptors are toxins that affect our genome and the function of our neurological, endocrine and immune systems. They have become ubiquitous in our environment. Many Endocrine Disruptors are also called persistent organic pollutants (POP's) because they resist environmental degradation and accumulate in animal fat cells. We then consume these animal products, whether we eat their meat or use dairy, and these POP's lodge in our bodies and our fat cells. We can also obtain POP's through consuming fruits, vegetables and grains.

An example of an Endocrine Disruptor affecting our human genome and causing disease concerns the epidemic of obesity and diabetes mellitus. The NHANES III study clearly showed that obesity does not cause diabetes mellitus. This runs contrary to everything that we have been taught over the past several decades. Yet, the study is very clear and definitive. In the NHANES III study, there was a correlation with GGT, a liver enzyme, and diabetes mellitus. When GGT was increased to the upper normal range or higher, patients had a very high likelihood of diabetes.

This was confirmed in studies on the western coast of Michigan where there is a very high rate of diabetes mellitus. The population was analyzed for risk factors for their diabetes, including their diet, and there were no risks factors identified that were any worse than other places in the United States. However, their GGT levels were higher than most other populations studied. GGT is a marker for glutathione depletion and exposure to POP's. In fact, when we look at the western coast of Michigan, they have extremely high levels of BPA in their bodies. This comes from Lake Michigan and all of the BPA that has been dumped into it on the Chicago side of the lake and has drifted over to the western shore of Michigan. People on the western shore typically are exposed to Lake Michigan water because they drink it and it is used to irrigate their crops. BPA poisons the mitochondria in our cells and results in an inability to manage sugar well, so we store it as fat. Thus, while obesity does not directly cause diabetes, it is a marker of toxin exposure and/or lifestyle risk factors.

What effects do Endocrine Disruptors have on our bodies?

- Increase or decrease hormone production
- Imitate hormones and increase their effects on the body
- Turn one hormone into another hormone entirely
- Interfere with hormone signaling, making it ineffective
- Binding to hormones to inactivate them
- Tell cells to die prematurely (Apoptosis)
- Decrease the absorption of nutrients
- Bind to nutrients to prevent their use by the body
- Suppress the immune system
- Interfere with the nervous system (Central and Peripheral)
- Cause cancers

Here are some examples of Endocrine Disruptors that we will look at in detail:

- Plastics
- Pesticides
- Pharmaceutical residue
- Herbicides
- Perchlorate
- PBDE's (polybrominated diphenyl ethers)
- Heavy metals (lead, mercury, and arsenic)
- PFC's (perflourinated chemicals)
- Solvents (glycol ethers)

PFH Action Point

- **Endocrine Disruptors are all around us and affect our genomic expression**
- **These include Persistent Organic Pollutants that may never degrade in the environment**
- **We must reduce our exposure to these toxins and get them out of our bodies**
- **They affect our neurological, endocrine, and immune systems**

Let's start by taking a look at plastics. If you were to start making a list of all of the plastic that you are exposed to on a daily basis, at the end of the day you would realize that you have hundreds of items on your list. Plastics are everywhere and are an unavoidable part of our daily life. What effect do these plastics have on our bodies?

The first plastic we will look at is Bisphenol A (BPA). BPA is toxic at very low doses to the human body. We commonly are exposed to BPA from plastics (polycarbonates) like #7 recycles. However, it is also in liquid infant formulas. BPA lines the cans of our fruits and vegetables, soups and drinks. It is found in baby bottles and food containers, such as the rigid plastic containers we use in our refrigerators and pantries.

It is very important that plastics containing BPA are not heated in any way, especially in the microwave. This releases the BPA into our food or beverages. We need to try to get all of the plastic out of our kitchen and away from our food. It should be noted that many manufacturers are cashing in on the public fears of BPA by marketing BPA-free plastics. These BPA-free containers are being made from other plastics that are just as toxic as BPA!

Ninety-three percent of Americans have BPA detectable in their bodies at potentially toxic levels. BPA is known to cause breast and prostate cancer, insulin resistance, obesity, heart disease, infertility, and PCOS (polycystic ovarian syndrome).

Another toxic plastic is PCB (polychlorinated biphenyl). PCB is a manmade chlorinated hydrocarbon that was banned in the United States in 1979. PCB is still present in old electric equipment and appliances, oil paints, caulk, and plastics that are in our landfills. The PCB then leaches out and gets into the water supply. PCB is highly concentrated in fish, especially fresh water fish. It is well known to cause cancers and neuro-endocrine-immune dysfunction.

Dioxin is another toxic plastic present in our environment. It is from the manufacture, molding, and burning of organic chemicals (pesticides, herbicides) and plastics that contain chlorine (PVC and chlorochemicals). Dioxin was also the major culprit in Agent Orange, which was used in Vietnam and contaminated some of our service men and women. Dioxin is also produced in paper mills when chlorine bleach is put on organic wood pulp. It is present in bleached coffee filters, #3 plastics, and all cling wraps.

Dioxin accumulates in fat cells including beef, pork, and fresh water fish. It also accumulates in milk and in full fat milk products (dairy). Dioxin causes cancers, birth defects, infertility, and neuro-endocrine-immune disorders. According to our government, most of the U.S. population has Dioxin present in their body at levels that can produce serious health effects.

Another plastic of great concern is phthalates. Phthalates are very common in our everyday lives and can go by the acronyms BDP, DEHP, BzBP, and DMP. Phthalates are very common in personal care products such as baby powders, shampoos, conditioners, and hair sprays. They are also common in flexible plastics including plastic wrap and plastic bags, which are commonly used for storage and heating of our foods. Phthalates are present in our cars, children's toys, and insect repellants. It can also be found on labels as "fragrance." Phthalates are typically found in #3 and #7 plastics. The health effects from phthalates are widespread. They disrupt the entire neuro-endocrine-immune system, and are responsible for many types of hormone imbalances. They also cause birth defects, obesity, diabetes, and thyroid disease. Once you start reading labels, you will see phthalates in most of your personal care products.

A specific phthalate worth mentioning is polyethylene terephthalate (PET), which is the predominant component in our plastic water bottles. The US consumes 30 billion plastic water bottles each year. That is 1500 every second. These bottles do not biodegrade, so they will exist in our landfills forever since only 2 in 10 will be recycled. As the water sits in these bottles in warm warehouses, hot transport trucks or our cars, phthalates leach into the water. These phthalates are ultimately consumed by us and lodge in our bodies to gradually poison us.

PFH Action Point

- **We must reduce our exposures to plastics in our food, water and personal care products**
- **Get the plastics out of the kitchen and never heat them**
- **Don't drink from plastic water bottles**
- **Read labels to find hidden phthalates**

All pesticides are potent Endocrine Disruptors. Most pesticides are related to organophosphates, created as chemical warfare agents in World War I and World War II. Now, they are used as insecticides all around us and on our food. Just because some insecticides, such as DDT, have been banned in the United States does not mean that they are not still being used in other countries. DDT was banned because of our Bald Eagles. DDT was found to weaken the shells of their eggs and they became nearly extinct. Since DDT was banned, our Bald Eagle has been making a comeback.

I live in Florida. There are bugs all around us. Pesticides are being sprayed routinely in our homes and on our lawns. We have golf courses everywhere and pesticides are used extensively on these golf courses. Our crops are being sprayed repeatedly with pesticides in an attempt to keep the bugs from destroying them. Pesticides then get into our water supply and food supply and into our bodies.

Pesticides affect brain development and behavior. Is it possible that some of the epidemic of ADD, ADHD, autism, and other behavioral disorders is due to the effects of pesticides? Pesticides also lower testosterone levels and directly affect testosterone function. They interfere with thyroid function. As with the Bald Eagles, they also lower fertility in human beings.

Pharmaceutical residues, from the manufacture of pharmaceuticals, also function as Endocrine Disruptors. These residues include chemotherapy agents, hormones, antibiotics, immune suppressants, and steroids. They contaminate our water supply and the air. Most filters do not remove them unless you are using a reverse osmosis system. These pharmaceutical residues can affect many organ systems, including the function of the hormone system, immune system, and GI tract.

Herbicides are used to control weeds and other unwanted vegetation. They have been very commonly used in our environment. We are all using them around our homes. Examples include atrazine, the second most widely used herbicide next to glyphosate (Roundup). Let's take a closer look at atrazine.

Seventy-six million pounds of atrazine are applied each year to U.S. food crops and to control unwanted vegetation. Atrazine has been banned in the European Union, but the FDA says it is perfectly safe for Americans. The company that makes atrazine, Syngenta, settled a 105 million dollar class action suit with municipal water supplies due to contamination of our drinking water. Atrazine contaminates most ground water in the United States. It is the most commonly detected pesticide/herbicide in U.S. drinking water. What does atrazine do to us? The most telling example is that atrazine turns male frogs into female frogs. It causes hormone disruption, breast tumors, prostate disease and cancers.

Perchlorate is the major component of rocket fuel. It contaminates our water supply, produce and milk products. How does rocket fuel get into our water, produce and milk? All of those jets flying through our skies on a daily basis leave perchlorate in our atmosphere. Rains then deposit it in our water supply and on our crops. Our animals eat and drink the perchlorate and then we eat them. Perchlorate interferes with iodine and results in thyroid hormone disruption. It also affects brain and other organ development in children.

BPDEs (polybrominated diphenyl ethers) are commonly used as fire retardants. You will find them in your foam furniture and carpet pads. They wind up in the dust in your home and settle on your furniture. We then breathe them in. BPDE levels in human breast milk are doubling every five years. They are found in almost all wildlife milk in the world. BPDEs disrupt thyroid hormone function by imitating its activity. It causes low IQ levels and other developmental brain disorders. You must be cautious and not reupholster old foam furniture. You also must be cautious replacing old carpeting, because the foam pad may have them. The only way to get them out of your home is to use a vacuum with a HEPA filter.

PFH Action Point

- **Get the pesticides off your food and out of your home**
- **Pharmaceutical residues and herbicides are in our water; use reverse osmosis water**
- **Perchlorate (rocket fuel) is in our water, produce and milk**
- **BPDE's (fire retardants) are in our home dust; be cautious redoing foam furniture and replacing carpet pads**

Endocrine Disruptors also include heavy metals. The first one we are going to look at is lead. Lead is well known to be especially toxic in children. However it is also toxic in adults. Lead is stored in bone and it is very hard to measure lead levels in the body. We try to approximate it by measuring blood samples of lead. This indicates a more current exposure. Chronic exposures need to be measured in other ways. Lead is present in older paints, drinking water and in cosmetics. It is scary to note that one of the largest sources of lead in cosmetics is lipstick. We will talk more about this later. Lead is also present in air pollution. For example, the pacific northwest of the United States has large amounts of lead in their air because of the burning of coal in China. Removing lead from gasoline has helped the United States air quality levels of lead somewhat, but now we are receiving lead in our air from other nations.

Lead causes brain damage and lowers IQ scores in both children and adults. It causes kidney and nervous system damage. Lead causes premature birth and miscarriages. It is also responsible for hypertension and hearing loss. Lead disrupts hormone signaling in the HPA (Hypothalamic Pituitary Adrenal) axis and our ability to deal with stress. Lead also significantly lowers sex hormones in men and women.

Another heavy metal of great concern is arsenic. Arsenic is not just a culprit in a who-done-it novel, but it is a culprit causing death in our real world. Large amounts of arsenic cause rapid death. Small amounts of arsenic cause a very slow death. Arsenic is present in our drinking water. It is also present in foods such as United States rice, apple juice and grape juice. Arsenic causes skin, bladder and lung cancers. It interferes with the function of our endocrine system. It is also responsible for osteoporosis, hypertension, insulin resistance (and diabetes mellitus), growth retardation, and immunosuppression.

Another heavy metal affecting our health is mercury. We are exposed to mercury in multiple different ways. Mercury is present in coal burning and so it is in the air that we breathe. This is especially true in New England and the Pacific Northwest. Because of the contamination of our air with mercury, it eventually winds up in our oceans and lakes. There it concentrates in fish, especially the larger predatory fish. These include tuna, swordfish, shark, mackerel, grouper, Chilean sea bass, and orange ruffy. There appears to be less mercury in salmon, trout, snapper, and mahi. Shrimp and scallops have very low levels.

Another source of mercury is dental amalgams. A typical dental amalgam filling will release one microgram of mercury each day into your body. If you have multiple fillings, such as I do, this can add up to a lot of mercury. Mercury interferes with fetal brain development, and therefore is a great concern for pregnant women. It interferes with hormone functions. Mercury damages pancreatic cells and can cause diabetes. It is also a cause of chronic fatigue.

PFH Action Point

- **Lead is in drinking water and cosmetics; it causes brain and other organ damage**
- **Arsenic is in drinking water, rice, apple and grape juice; it causes cancer and other diseases**
- **Mercury is in fish and dental amalgams; it causes fatigue, hormone disruption, diabetes**
- **Reverse Osmosis water filtration will remove these**
- **No more domestic rice or rice products, apple or grape juice**

PFC's (Perflourochemicals) are present in our homes in several ways. They are the main component in nonstick cookware. Over time, they leach out into the foods we are preparing and lodge in our bodies. PFC's are also present in water resistant coatings on clothing, furniture, and carpets. Since our children are usually on the floor or on our furniture at very young ages, with their faces in these things, this is of great concern. Ninety-nine percent of the U.S. population has PFC's in their bodies. PFC's will never degrade in the environment and will persist for generations. They cause thyroid and kidney disease, low birth weights, and sex hormone disruption.

Solvents are also common and we are exposed to them on a daily basis. We are not just talking about workers who are using these products. Solvents are present in paints, cleaning products, brake fluid and cosmetics. An example of a toxic solvent is glycol ether. It is hard to believe that these solvents are in your cosmetics, but they are. What do they do? Solvents result in decreased fertility, blood abnormalities, asthma, and allergies.

Another chemical of concern is nonylphenol, which results from the breakdown of nonionic surfactants that are widely used in home and industry. Products containing these chemicals include detergents, paints, personal care products and plastics. It is produced during wastewater transport and treatment and has accumulated in the environment. It contaminates ground water and fresh water bodies, resulting in fish being contaminated, as well. Nonylphenol is a POP and an Endocrine Disruptor and appears on the Dirty Dozen list of chemicals that result in cancer.

VOC's (Volatile Organic Compounds) are becoming more well-known and their effects more documented and studied. VOC's are present in floor and wall coverings, particle board, adhesives, and paints. They are also present as toxic benzene derivatives in disinfectants and deodorizers. New carpeting releases several of these VOC's and it can take many months for them to "off gas" to safer levels. The VOC's in carpeting also trap pesticides at high levels.

Other types of VOC's include those compounds and toxins released by toxic mold and the other contaminants in the interior of Water Damaged Buildings (WDB's) into the air. Mycotoxins can also be carried on other chemicals in the air that enable them to enter your Respiratory System easier. We will examine Mycotoxins and the other toxins inside WDB's later.

VOC's cause kidney damage, immune dysfunction, hormone imbalance, blood disorders, asthma, and bronchitis. How can we deal with these VOC's? The best thing to do is to eliminate carpet or to air out the home after installation for several months. We need to start using VOC-free cleaners and low-VOC paints. Air purifiers that are certified to remove VOC's are also helpful. We need to get toxic mold and other contaminants of WDB's out of our homes. This requires a careful search and remediation by specialists.

PFH Action Point

- **PFC's are in our homes; stop using non-stick cookware and water resistant coatings**
- **Solvents are in cosmetics, paints and cleaning products; they cause asthma and blood abnormalities**
- **Nonylphenol results from the chemicals in detergents, paints, personal care products and plastics; it is an Endocrine Disruptor and causes cancer**
- **VOC's are in our homes; get rid of carpet, use VOC-free cleaners and consider using a HEPA/VOC air purifier; Search for toxic mold and eliminate it**

Personal care products are a big source of Endocrine Disruptors for all of us. This includes shampoo, conditioner, hair sprays, coloring agents, straightening agents, cosmetics, skin care products, and sunscreens. This also includes baby powders and lotions. These personal care products are loaded with Endocrine Disruptors like phthalates, toxic chemicals like glycol ethers, heavy metals, dyes, and fragrances. The average woman puts 16 different products on herself every morning with over 10 ingredients in each one. That means 160 potentially toxic chemicals every morning. The average woman eats 6 pounds of lipstick in her lifetime. Most of this lipstick contains lead. Thinking about that should make you feel ill and not want to use lipstick ever again.

Another ingredient in personal care products that should concern us is triclosan. It is a prominent ingredient in liquid hand soaps, dishwashing liquids and personal care products. It is an antibacterial and antifungal agent, so it appears often in "antibacterial" products. It is also used in toothbrushes, toys and cutting boards. Triclosan is an Endocrine Disruptor and is toxic to several organ systems. It frequently causes allergic reactions on the skin and in the eyes. Its use results in the development of resistant bacteria and fungi, a major problem. It is on the Dirty Dozen list of chemicals to avoid to prevent cancer.

There are approximately 85,000 registered chemicals in the United States. Ninety percent of these chemicals have never been tested for human health effects or toxicity. Manufacturers can use almost any ingredient they choose without having to supply safety data. The FDA can't require safety tests or recall harmful products. Thus, our personal care products are loaded with chemicals that have never been tested for human safety and are potentially hazardous.

A good resource for chemical safety is on the Environmental Working Group website (ewg.org). The Skin Deep database contains about 85,000 products with ratings on toxicity and potential health effects. You can even get an app for your phone. Check out your personal care products and see where they stand. If they are not rated well, change to something else. Beware of organic personal care products. Read the ingredient list very carefully. Just because something is labeled "organic", does not mean it can't contain one or more toxic chemicals.

PFH Action Point

- **Personal Care Products are a big source of Endocrine Disruptors like phthalates, toxic chemicals, heavy metals, triclosan, dyes and fragrances**
- **There are minimal safety standards for these products**
- **You must read labels and eliminate toxins yourself**
- **Check the Skin Deep database at Environmental Working Group for help in choosing the right products**

5. EMF

EMF is the term used for Electromagnetic Field (electrosmog) exposure. While there has been a lot of media attention given to cell phones, it is much more than just that. Regarding cell phones, if you start using one as a teenager, you have five times the risk of brain cancer as those who started using them as an adult. This is very concerning. EMF is the chronic exposure to low-level radiation. It can cause cancers, heart disease, impaired immunity, sleep disorders, hormone imbalances, and contribute to dementia. This EMF can also come from so-called dirty electricity (very low frequency voltage) from electronics and appliances. This dirty electricity increases the risk of cancers, including melanoma, thyroid, and uterine cancer.

EMF disrupts brain waves and causes behavioral problems. It interferes with cellular communication and may cause neurological disorders such as Autism and Alzheimer's dementia. EMF changes the cell membrane to impermeable so that Free Radicals accumulate within the cell and cause more damage. This results in damage to DNA and prevents DNA repair.

What can we do to prevent EMF exposure and potential damage? We can try to use laptops on battery power only because the charger is a bad source of EMF. We can try to avoid cell phone towers, microwave dishes, and power lines. We should only use our cell phone when we have the maximum number of bars; otherwise, the cell phone is generating more EMF to try to reach a distant tower. We should also not use our cell phone in a car, train, plane, or metal building as this will increase our EMF exposure. Experts recommend eliminating the following: microwave ovens, plasma televisions, electric blankets/heating pads, cordless phones, wifi, Bluetooth, the location transmitter on cell phones, tablets, laptops, devices that repel insects/animals, location transmitters in appliances and electronics (hidden), and fluorescent lights.

Given our ubiquitous exposure to EMF in our daily environments, what can we do to reduce its effect or treat its damage? Probiotics reduce electrosensitivity. We will talk more about probiotics later. Detoxification of toxic organisms also helps because EMF increases toxic production. One example is the need to eliminate toxic mold if you are genetically susceptible to it. EMF will increase neurotoxin production by toxic mold by 600 times!

It is important in EMF treatment to create a sleep sanctuary as EMF also interferes with sleep. Some things that can be done include using only a battery clock near the bed and not an electric clock; unplugging electric devices in the bedroom; eliminating radiofrequency signals from portable phones, cell phones and wireless devices in the bedroom; and using a bed without metal.

PFH Action Point
- **EMF (electrosmog) is a real danger to your health**
- **It affects your brain waves, causes behavioral and neurological disorders, and increases cancer risk**
- **It is essential to limit your EMF exposure to cell phones, power lines, cell towers and microwave dishes; construct a safe bedroom environment**
- **Probiotics reduce electrosensitivity; detoxification of toxin producing organisms is important as EMF increases toxin production**

6. Biotoxins

One of the next big waves getting ready to break in medicine is the subject of Biotoxins. Biotoxins are organisms that cause a condition called Chronic Inflammatory Response Syndrome (CIRS). The organisms include toxic mold (there are at least five of them that cause this disorder), Lyme disease, Ciguatera fish poisoning, Brown Recluse spider bites, and Pfisteria. The result is an immune system that is chronically inflamed and this causes a host of diseases and symptoms. Unless the chronic **inflammation** is corrected, the diseases and symptoms never go away.

The opportunity to get a CIRS is dependent on your genetic makeup. Twenty-four percent of the U.S. population has the genetics to get toxic mold illness. Since NIOSH says that fifty percent of the buildings in the United States are water damaged (WDB's), and any of these could have toxic mold, there is a big reservoir for exposure. That also means that seventy-six percent of the population cannot get toxic mold illness. This is why a hundred people can be in a sick building and only 24 or less will get sick. Along the same lines, twenty percent of the U.S. population has the genetics to acquire Chronic Lyme disease if exposed to the bite of a deer tick in an endemic area. That means that eighty percent of the population cannot get Chronic Lyme disease from a tick bite.

Why has this happened to us? Prior to the 1970's, we were building homes differently. They "breathed" more and outside air was able to dilute the inside air in our homes and offices. We kept the windows open and had fans on to bring in outside air. The same was true for our cars. Everyone drove around with the windows open. Then we began to get energy efficient in the construction of our homes. Much of this was under federal direction due to the stranglehold on our nation from foreign oil producers in the 1970's. We tightened everything up in the construction of our homes to make the structures energy efficient and air was not able to get in any more. We started using thick insulation and drywall instead of plaster. By the way, drywall, when it gets wet, is the perfect medium for mold growth. Nothing could grow on the plaster. Mold remediation professionals know that once the drywall and carpet get wet, they have very little time to get it all removed before the mold starts to grow. Generally, this is less than 48 hours.

At the same time, we started installing central HVAC systems, which stands for Heating/Ventilation/Air Conditioning. That meant we needed to keep the doors and windows closed. We started putting AC systems in our cars and closed those windows also. Now, we go from one HVAC system to another throughout our day to keep a comfortable temperature. All the time, we are breathing in re-circulated air. The same happens when you take an airplane trip; you are concerned about the re-circulated air on the plane and the risk for infections, but what about in your home and workplace? Think how tightly the typical office building is constructed and how susceptible it is to contamination when there is water damage. The average American is breathing indoor air for 94% of the day, most of which is re-circulated and potentially contaminated.

I have learned a lot about HVAC systems from an HVAC and indoor air specialist God introduced me to. He has shown me how many HVAC systems have had their outside air returns closed down by HVAC contractors and maintenance people so that they can cool better. This is a huge mistake and results in the system being starved for air return and re-circulating inside air. The result is that it will develop poor seals around the air handler and begin to suck in air from the attic or wherever the air handler is located. Imagine what is in that air. The unit runs too cold and moisture develops, resulting in the perfect breeding environment for mold. Once the air handler is contaminated, the entire building becomes infected.

Once the structure is contaminated by mold, either through water damage or a contaminated HVAC system, the potential for sickness is present. The mold spores, once they are exposed to water, release substances called mycotoxins. They also release these when they die and break apart and when they enter the human body and deposit on the moist lining of your respiratory tract. These mycotoxins are now in the air, on the flooring, on the surfaces, in your clothes, and on the furniture. Since the air is re-circulated and the building is so tightly constructed, the concentration of mycotoxins increases. Elevated humidity levels, above 62%, further encourage mold growth. The concentration of mycotoxins in the air can determine how quickly and severely you react. The mold spores and the mycotoxins get into your body and wreak havoc with your immune system.

Those with the genetic susceptibility for toxic mold illness or Chronic Lyme disease have a specific genetic defect on chromosome 6. Major laboratories can test for these genetic sequences easily. If you have one of these genetic types, then you cannot process toxic mold organisms, or the organism that causes Lyme disease, once they enter your body. The result is an inability to make antibodies to kill the organism. The organism secretes a mycotoxin (neurotoxin) that binds to your central nervous system and begins to wreak havoc on your body's immune system. The immune system becomes chronically inflamed because it cannot fight off these invaders, but it keeps on trying 24 hours a day, 365 days a year. The inflammatory substances called Cytokines that are released by our bodies result in multiple hormone abnormalities in the brain and elsewhere. The immune compromise results in many different infections, including antibiotic resistant staph in the sinuses.

The symptoms of CIRS include fatigue, pain, headaches, gut problems, cognitive and memory problems, and strange neurological symptoms. CIRS looks a lot like Fibromyalgia, Chronic Fatigue and Immune Dysfunction Syndrome, Thyroid and Adrenal Disease, and Autoimmune Disorders. In children, CIRS often looks like ADHD, Autism, and vague complaints. Chronic **inflammation** leads to a host of other diseases.

There is a great screening test for CIRS. It is found on survivingmold.com, the website of Dr. Ritchie Shoemaker, who I consider to be the leading expert on CIRS. It is called the VCS test; it stands for Visual Contrast Sensitivity test. The VCS test was developed by the U.S. military to use in testing fighter pilots. However, Dr. Shoemaker discovered that it is an effective screening tool for patients with CIRS. There are specific instructions on how to take the VCS test online. If you have the symptoms of CIRS and fail the VCS test, then there is a 98.5% chance that you have CIRS. There is a small percentage of patients that can pass the VCS test and still have this disorder. You can learn a lot more about CIRS at survivingmold.com.

In my private medical practice, I am caring for a number of patients with CIRS. Most have been misdiagnosed for years as having Fibromyalgia, Chronic Fatigue Syndrome, or numerous other chronic disorders. Most have been labeled as depressed, anxious, or having other psychological impairments. Misdiagnosis is the rule rather than the exception in this condition. Normal laboratory testing does not reveal the immune system abnormalities. Most patients are thought to be crazy by their physicians and healthcare practitioners.

CIRS patients undergo extensive laboratory evaluation, including genetic testing and assessment of the immune system, hormone system, and thyroid and adrenal systems. There is a complex detoxification regimen that, if done correctly, results in a cure. If the inflamed immune system does not correct on its own, there are steps to restore regulation. I follow Dr. Shoemaker's protocols exactly since he has the most experience in the world treating these patients. Patients must be removed from exposures to water damaged buildings in order to heal. This often means remediating their home or leaving it entirely.

It also means assessing the workplace and other buildings where they spend a lot of time. Patients have to be taught how to avoid further exposures and what to do when one happens. Could your home and buildings be making you sick?

PFH Action Point

- **Biotoxin Illness is emerging as a major health threat**
- **It looks like Fibromyalgia, Chronic Fatigue Syndrome, and other chronic vague ills**
- **Causes include toxic mold from water damaged buildings and Chronic Lyme Disease**
- **The VCS test at survivingmold.com is a great screening test**

- **Treatment includes removing yourself from exposure, detoxification, and restoring regulation to the inflamed immune system**

Mycotoxins are those substances released from fungi to destroy their hosts and allow them to penetrate and grow in them. Most work to impair and eventually damage our immune systems. These fungi are not just present in WDB's. They are also present in our food supply.

Mycotoxins have been around a long time and some have been found useful. For example, penicillin is actually a mycotoxin from the Penicillium mold discovered by Fleming. Mycotoxins will actually kill bacteria so the fungi can grow and eat whatever it is growing on without having to share it. They have been used in many medications, including antibiotics and immune suppressing agents, and unfortunately, as chemical warfare agents. The US used a mycotoxin in Vietnam.

The most deadly toxin of any kind for humans, in the world, is Aflatoxin B1, which is made by the mold Aspergillus. It was first discovered in London in 1962 when ground peanut meal was found to have caused 100,000 turkey deaths. Zearalenone, which is made by Fusarium, is very estrogenic, making it an Endocrine Disruptor and it causes tremendous problems for women, including premature puberty. Fusarium contamination has been a problem with contact lens solutions. Penicillium produces a tremorgenic mycotoxin, which, as the name implies, causes tremors in humans. Stachybotrys produces Trichochecenes, a well-studied mycotoxin with numerous health effects.

Mycotoxins have been shown to cause numerous cancers—Kidney, Esophagus, Liver, Testicles, Prostate, Leukemia. They have also been linked to respiratory problems like asthma and bronchitis and bone marrow and immune system suppression. Mycotoxins have been associated with childhood intellectual decline and behavioral disorders. Trichochecenes, in particular, has been shown to affect the brain and neurologic system, immune system, heart, lungs, intestines, liver, kidney and skin. The CDC and NIH lists it as a potent toxin with numerous serious health effects and potentially causing death.

Mycotoxins are a major problem in our food supply, especially in grains. Just think about it. You have a silo full of wheat, which is basically a carbohydrate (sugar), which is the perfect medium for mold growth. Add a little humidity or water, and you have contaminated wheat. In fact, this happens with corn, wheat, barley, rye, sorghum, and cottonseed. Corn is heavily contaminated with mycotoxins such as Fumonisin, Aflatoxin, Zearalenone, and Ochratoxin. Wheat is also heavily contaminated and so are all of the products made from wheat. Is gluten sensitivity really a reaction to the mycotoxins?

The American Food and Agriculture Organization estimates that 25% of the world's food crops are affected by mycotoxins. Once the grains are contaminated, so is the rest of the food chain that eats them. Think of all the grain-fed animals and animal products we consume, such as meat, eggs and dairy products. We are the final stop in the food chain and are accumulating all those mycotoxins in our bodies.

Other products that are potentially contaminated with mycotoxins include alcoholic beverages, because they are made from grains and other contaminated products. In fact, the alcohol is a mycotoxin produced by Saccharomyces yeast (brewer's yeast). Sugar beets and sugar cane are also potentially contaminated; fungi like sugar as much as we do. Peanuts can be very badly contaminated and have been found in one study to have 24 different types of fungi inside the shell. Hard cheeses can easily grow mold that produce mycotoxins. Remember that citric acid is made as a mycotoxin and appears in many processed foods.

There are some natural treatments for mycotoxins that will help you and your family to avoid toxicity. First and foremost, remove yourself from the exposure. If you are living in a mold contaminated structure, get out and get it remediated. If you are being exposed from your foods, eliminate them. Try to eat as few of the mentioned grains as possible. Avoid sugar from sugar cane and sugar beets (many of which are GMO anyway). It is best to eliminate corn and corn products (remember, they are mostly GMO also unless organic). Avoid alcoholic beverages as they are made from grains and products contaminated with mycotoxins (and alcohol is a toxin anyway). Avoid eating peanuts and peanut products, like peanut butter. Limit hard cheeses and avoid them if you see any mold growth.

Probiotics will help to repopulate your digestive tract with good bacteria and help maintain a good balance of defense against fungi and other foreign invaders. We will discuss what to look for in a Probiotic later. Consume organic produce and herbs that help to fight mold, including carrots, kale, garlic, ginger, cayenne, and oregano. In fact, oregano oil has mold-killing properties.

PFH Action Point

- **Mycotoxins are produced from a wide range of mold and include Aflatoxin, Zearalenone, and Trichothecenes**
- **Some are deadly and others are immune suppressants and Endocrine Disruptors**
- **Mycotoxins contaminate up to 25% of the world's food crops, including many grains**
- **Avoid alcoholic beverages, wheat, corn, many grains, sugar, peanuts; limit hard cheeses**
- **Some natural treatments include herbs and produce, Probiotics, and oregano oil**

In summary, we are living in a very toxic environment and our health is being threatened at multiple points every day. We are the main ingredients in a toxic soup! It is only by the grace of God that we, and our children, will survive. While the Lord is longsuffering, I am not sure how long He will continue to let us ruin His creation. There is coming a time, very soon, when Jesus will return and our planet will be remade into an unpolluted Garden of Eden. Until then, you must take steps today to protect your health and the health of your family.

Chapter 6
Your Prescription for Health

As we start the journey together into better health for you and your family, let us first take a few moments to review what we have already discussed.

We started our journey by first taking a look at the health care problems that we are facing in our nation. We examined the explosion of chronic diseases that are affecting our health and vitality. Vague problems such as fatigue, generalized pain, depression, anxiety, gut problems, headaches and hormone imbalances are prevalent throughout our society. Our government, the healthcare system, and the medical establishment have been unable to deal with the diseases that we face and the symptoms that we are dealing with on a daily basis. I presented the possibility that there was a conspiracy behind our health dilemmas and that we were going to have to take individual action for our health and the health of our families.

We discussed how **inflammation** is the bottom line of the diagnosis inverted-pyramid. The causes of our **inflammation** include Free Radicals, nutrient deficiencies, food chain toxins, environmental toxins, and Biotoxins. We have reviewed in detail the toxic world that we are living in and the tremendous challenges that we are facing. At the conclusion of the last chapter, you were probably thinking that this is totally hopeless. You probably thought that things are only going to get worse, so why even try to get healthy?

There is hope. If we can adopt an **anti-inflammatory lifestyle**, then we cannot only survive in this toxic world, but we can flourish.

Physicians typically spend a large portion of their day writing prescriptions. These prescriptions are often potentially toxic pharmaceuticals with numerous side effects. As a Functional Medicine physician, I try to write very few of these. Instead, I prescribe natural therapies to help restore the balance to our physical bodies. I also address the emotional and spiritual lives of my patients. It is only through this holistic approach that we can hope to feel truly well. I am writing for you a *Prescription for Health*. If you choose to fill the prescription, you will be healthier and feel better. As with any prescription, the choice to fill it is yours.

Mankind has always been given the ability to freely choose what to do. In the Garden of Eden, God gave Adam and Eve the ability to choose. Many people ask me why God did this in the first place. Why didn't God just program us to obey Him? My answer is pretty simple. God does not want to force us to love Him. What pleasure is there in that? God desires that we choose to love Him because we want to. He desires that we choose to obey Him because it is the best thing for us. Adam and Eve chose to disobey God, and eat of the tree of the knowledge of good and evil, and the consequences of that decision have plagued humanity since that time.

Again we are faced with a critical choice. Are we going to continue to do the same things that have gotten us into this healthcare crisis, expecting that somehow things will get better, or are we going to choose to change? Einstein's definition of insanity is to do the same things over and over again expecting different results. The Bible has a term for people who choose to do that. In Proverbs, Solomon calls those kinds of people fools. Wise people are portrayed as those who see the problems they are facing and make a course correction to go in a different way to either avoid those problems or to correct them. I don't know about you, but I don't want to be a fool. I would much prefer to be a wise person.

In order to repair the damage that has been done to our bodies, we are going to have to choose to make some changes. Actually, these changes are fairly significant. We can no longer listen to what the government, its bureaucratic agencies, the medical establishment, pharmaceutical companies, big agriculture companies, chemical companies, and the media are telling us to do. We must examine the scientific evidence for ourselves and make our own decisions.

When a new patient comes to my medical practice, I typically spend an hour with them reviewing their history, symptoms, and prior evaluations and treatments. I ask them a lot of questions and try to play the role of the medical detective, using our diagnosis inverted-pyramid, to arrive at the bottom line: the diagnosis of what is wrong with them. I then will do a physical examination and order extensive laboratory evaluations to rule out or confirm the diagnosis. Before they go, I give the patient a handout explaining what is wrong with them and how their life has gotten out of balance. I tell them that we are going to have to work on many issues to restore the balance to their life. These include nutrition, nutrient deficiencies, toxins, endocrine imbalances, sleep dysfunction, stress, exercise/physical activity, and their spiritual life. Only when we restore the balance in all of these areas, will the patient actually feel better.

I also give the patient a list of homework assignments that they must complete before their next visit. These are some simple but difficult changes that they need to start making in their life. When they return for their second visit, typically to review all of their laboratory findings, I ask how they did with their homework assignments. Some patients are very motivated and have completed all of them. Some patients are overwhelmed and have only completed a few. Some patients, unfortunately, have not completed any of them and don't seem very motivated to try. These patients are still living in the traditional medical world where they could get a pill for their problem and not have to change anything in their life. I tell them that none of their problems will get better with a pill or they would have already found results. I explain to them that if they are not willing to make the needed changes in their life, then they could expect to get worse over time. I also tell them that if they are not willing to follow my instructions, that this is probably not the right medical practice for them to be in.

I am assuming that if you are reading this book that you have some desire to get healthy. Hopefully, you now understand that this is going to take some work on your part. I will provide you with the information and guidance that you need to know what changes to make. However, I can't be with you 24/7; you have to decide that change is important and that you are going to take responsibility for your healthcare.

During my second visit, I give the patient another handout that is my general treatment plan that they are to follow. It contains a lot of information. I will be including all of that in subsequent chapters and going into greater detail than I can during an office visit. If you take a look at the treatment pyramid in this book, you will get a general sense of what we will be discussing. We will be examining each of these items in greater detail.

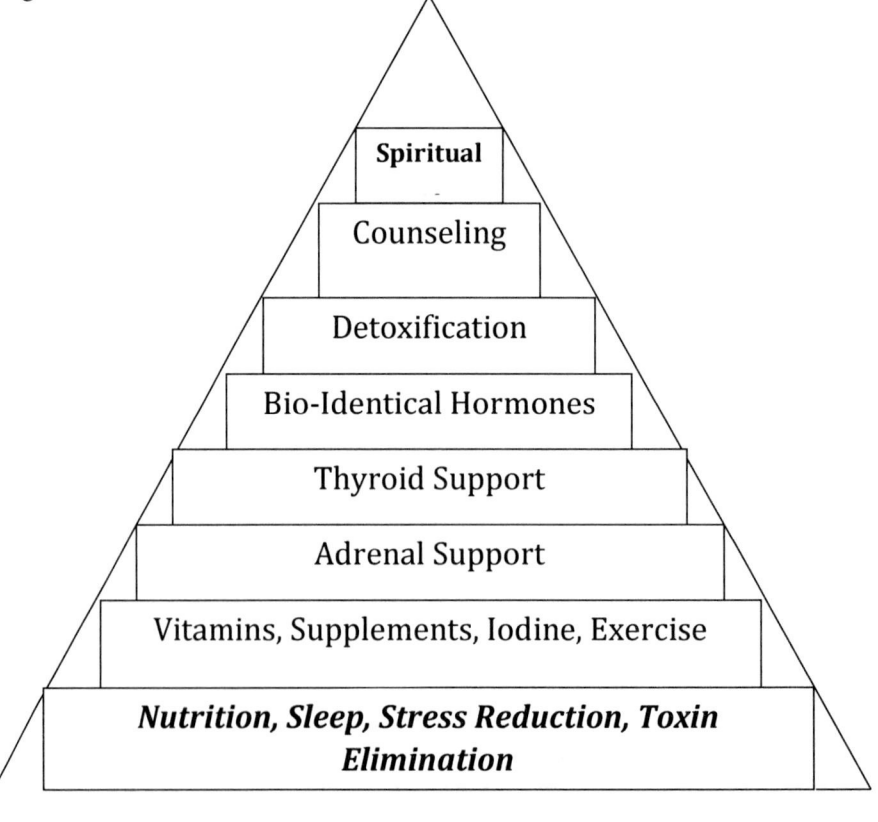

```
                    Spiritual
                   Counseling
                 Detoxification
              Bio-Identical Hormones
                Thyroid Support
                Adrenal Support
        Vitamins, Supplements, Iodine, Exercise
    Nutrition, Sleep, Stress Reduction, Toxin
                   Elimination
```

I want you to notice that the cornerstone of the treatment pyramid is nutrition. Just as Christ is the cornerstone of the Church, so nutrition is the cornerstone of our **anti-inflammatory lifestyle**. Just as without Christ the entire Church would collapse, so it is with nutrition. Without making changes in your nutritional program, the rest of the pyramid will collapse and you will not be successful.

How you choose to implement the changes we will be discussing is up to you. Some people, like me, prefer to make the changes all at once. Some of my patients, like me, find it less painful to just get it all over with instead of dragging the process out. Some people prefer to go more slowly and to make gradual changes over a longer period of time. Whatever you decide to do to implement our **anti-inflammatory lifestyle**, my advice to you is to set a goal and just do it.

I don't know how many of you have seen the movie "What About Bob?" If you haven't, I highly suggest that you watch it. The movie is hysterical. One of the memorable parts of the movie is Bob getting advice from his psychiatrist to make changes by taking baby steps. This means starting with just one little step forward and then taking another little step forward. If you continue to do that, eventually you will get to your goal. If that is how you would prefer to implement our **anti-inflammatory lifestyle**, that is great. Perhaps consider watching this movie, as it will greatly relieve your stress. Laughter is a good thing for the immune system.

Invariably, you will fail. It is not a matter of if, but a matter of when. Your failure may be something small, such as eating the wrong thing when you go out to dinner, or it can be something big, such as going off our **anti-inflammatory lifestyle** entirely. The Bible says that the same thing happens with sin. Invariably, we will mess up and fall into some type of sin. However, 1 John 1:9 says that if we confess our sins, God is faithful and just to forgive us of our sins and to cleanse us of all unrighteousness. This means that we get another chance.

If you fail at something we will be discussing, then just commit to start again. This is like falling off a bicycle. The best thing to do is to wipe yourself off, gather yourself, and get back on the bicycle and ride again. The main thing is to not give up. There is too much at stake here.

Your future quality of life, and the quality of the lives of your family members, is dependent on you making these changes and sticking with them. Failure is not an option. There is a word in the Bible called perseverance. The definition of perseverance is quite interesting. While many people use it interchangeably with patience, they are not the same words. Perseverance is the ability to be patient under affliction or trials, but not to just endure it. It is the decision that you are going to grow despite the difficulties. Perseverance means to make a conscious choice to put up with the pain and become better for it. That is what I want you to do here - make the changes that we will be discussing, put up with doing it, and be determined to come out better for it.

So, let's begin our journey together.

PFH Action Point

- **Adopt an anti-inflammatory lifestyle.**
- **Either take baby steps or just do it all at once.**
- **When you fail, just start again – don't give up!**
- **There is a lot at stake – your future quality of life.**

Chapter 7
EAT TO LIVE!

The cornerstone of our treatment pyramid, which I revealed to you in the last chapter, and our **anti-inflammatory lifestyle** is nutrition. None of you will get well without changing the way you eat. I have been dealing with very sick, complex medical patients for over ten years utilizing a holistic treatment program. I can assure you that none of my patients have ever gotten well without changing the way they eat. In many cases this means a radical change. For some of you, this may only mean minor changes in what you are currently doing. I encourage you to go into this with an open mind.

We all need to adopt a new paradigm in this country. We need to eat to live <u>not</u> live to eat. In America, we have equated prosperity and a higher standard of living with eating more and more food. It seems that much of our time is devoted to living to eat. We cook elaborate meals and go out to restaurants and fast food establishments and seem to devote a large amount of time to eating. While there is a lot of social interaction and pleasure that can occur with eating, the main purpose for our taking in nutrition is not those things. We should be eating in order to nourish our bodies, allowing for repair and healing. We should be recharging our antioxidant defense mechanisms and detoxification pathways. We should be preventing and fighting off diseases and infections. We should be trying to strive for a better quality of life versus a larger quantity of life.

This paradigm switch will require behavioral and cultural changes. We have all been brought up a certain way and have been conditioned to do certain things by our government, families, schools, and media. The misinformation that we have been given all of our lives has made us who we are. We all have to decide to change. Change is hard, but it will be well worth it.

As we begin to look at nutrition as the cornerstone of our **anti-inflammatory lifestyle**, the first paradigm shift that we have to make is this idea of eating three meals a day. I want to stress to you how important it is to balance your blood sugars. Eating three meals a day will result in large fluctuations in your blood sugars throughout the day. This results in stress on your pancreas, adrenal and thyroid glands. All of these organs have some role to play in balancing your blood sugars. There is a complex interaction between insulin, Cortisol and thyroid hormone. The more that we can keep these hormones at steady states in your body, the more efficiently you will burn sugar as energy and not store it as fat.

In order to balance your blood sugars, you need to try to eat three meals and three snacks daily. Thus, you're trying to eat something every two to three hours. These do not have to be large meals. In fact, we want to try to restrict our calorie consumption as studies clearly show that the more calories we eat, the more diseases we develop. This is not just restricted to obesity and diabetes. We now know that excess calories result in certain type of cancers, chromosome damage, and shortened life spans.

Each of our meals should have a high quality protein, high quality fats, and fiber. How much protein you need per day is dependent upon your height, weight, body mass index (BMI) and activity level. In general, it is not necessary for most of us to have more than 15 to 20 grams of protein at each meal. Americans eat far too much protein compared to other cultures in the world. We should be focusing on eating fruits, vegetables, protein, nuts, seeds, beans, and lentils. We will look in more detail at these later. We need to limit starches, sugar, and other bad carbohydrates, including most grains.

PFH Action Point

- **Nutrition is the cornerstone of our treatment pyramid**
- **You will not get well without changing the way you eat**
- **Eat to live, not live to eat**
- **Balance blood sugars by eating 3 meals and 3 snacks daily**

Snacks can be something simple such as a handful of nuts or a small piece of fruit. Snacks are not meant to be large meals. The purpose of a snack is again to try to keep your blood sugar at a steady level throughout the day. A snack can include things such as hummus, salsa, avocados, or guacamole on a piece of vegetable or a gluten free, rice free organic cracker or chip. At this point patients often ask me what in the world they can actually eat. I try to keep it simple for them and I hopefully can keep it simple for you.

What I am asking you to do is to eat a diet that consists of whole foods. There are many different variations of this diet out there on the market, but again I prefer to keep it simple. If we can eat foods that are in their natural state, created by God in their raw form, we will be doing pretty well. What I am advising is eliminating most processed foods, which includes anything with an ingredient list. The more ingredients a food product has, the more potential for toxic exposure. It is best to just eliminate foods with an ingredient list entirely.

So what do we do for snacks then? Certainly it is ok to have some snack foods that have a limited ingredient list. For example, I like organic salsa or guacamole on tortilla chips. Most tortilla chips are made with genetically modified corn and rancid oils. However, it is very easy now to find organic blue corn tortilla chips that are non-GMO and made with expeller pressed organic oils that are not GMO. The ingredient list only contains three things: organic corn, oil, and sea salt. This would be something safe to have. While it would be best to make your own tortilla chips, this is not practical for most of us. There are other chips that are made from non-GMO ingredients that are organic and can be healthy, including organic potato, black bean, and other vegetable chips. Beware of organic chips or crackers made with rice as the Arsenic concern is still present, organic or not. Obviously, wheat crackers are off limits.

Let's look at popcorn for example. In the old days, people used to pop their own corn on the stove top using a metal pan and some oil. Then came along air poppers and finally the microwave popcorn that we have become used to today. Microwave popcorn is a definite snack to avoid. There are numerous toxins in microwave popcorn and the employees that work at the plants producing these things have extremely high rates of cancer. They contain fake butter and other bad fats. How could real butter be dried up in a bag for months and be any good for you? Do you really want to eat that? An alternative would be to get a stainless steel popcorn popper to use on top of the stove with an organic cooking oil that has a high flash point. You can easily purchase organic popping corn, certified non-GMO, and make your own, seasoning it to taste. You can even use real organic butter if you want!

PFH Action Point

- **Snacks are a small piece of fruit or a dozen nuts**
- **Salsa or guacamole on a veggie or organic tortilla chip**
- **Avoid chips and crackers made from wheat or rice**
- **Don't eat microwave popcorn-make your own organic popcorn on the stove top**

In this new, **anti-inflammatory lifestyle**, we need to be focusing our attention on consuming fresh fruits and vegetables. Given the many problems we identified previously with the food chain, and the toxins that can potentially contaminate our produce, it is very important to know the source of your fruits and vegetables. It is always best to obtain your produce locally, buying it as close to the time it was picked as possible. If you have the time and desire to do so, growing your own organic produce would be the best thing. While the food industry may criticize organic produce and claim that it is not much different than nonorganic produce, the facts are clearly different. Organic produce is generally free of toxic pesticides and is grown in soil that contains more nutrients. Studies show that organic produce has approximately 25% more vitamins and minerals than regular produce. This is very significant.

In our quest to bolster our immune system, specifically our antioxidant defense system against Free Radicals, it is important to consume a large variety of fruits and vegetables. While some antioxidants are generated within our cells, specifically glutathione, most of our antioxidants come from external sources. You may have heard the term "rainbow color of produce." This refers to the recommendation from experts that we consume fruits and vegetables of many different colors in order to obtain the antioxidants and other nutrients that our bodies need. This produce includes both dark, leafy green vegetables and more brightly colored fruits and vegetables. Don't forget about dark blues and purples because they contain some of the highest concentrations of antioxidants.

While it is best to eat fruits and vegetables raw, vegetables can be lightly steamed or lightly sautéed without harming too many of the nutrients. Many antioxidants are very heat sensitive and so significant cooking of fruits and vegetables will destroy much of their enzyme activity and antioxidants. Some vegetables, such as cruciferous vegetables (broccoli, cauliflower, kale, and brussels sprouts) will actually contain similar amounts of antioxidants from lightly cooking them, but thyroid-interfering chemicals will be significantly reduced.

Given the higher cost of organic produce in general, it may not be possible for you to eat totally organic fruits and vegetables. Is there a guide to help us understand which ones are essential to purchase organic? Yes, fortunately there is. The Environmental Working Group publishes yearly lists called the Dirty Dozen and the Clean 15. You can find them on their website ewg.org and you can even get an app for your phone, so that you can refer to these lists while you are in the supermarket. The Dirty Dozen are the fruits and vegetables that you absolutely must eat organic; they are contaminated with too many pesticides and it is very difficult to wash them off. The Clean 15 is a list of those fruits and vegetables that you may be able to buy in a non-organic form. Generally these are things that you can peel. Please note that these lists do not take into account the higher nutrient levels present in organic produce. This is just taking into account residual pesticide levels found on produce in supermarkets throughout the United States.

For those of you who want to find a way to decontaminate your fruits and vegetables from any potential pesticides and bacteria, there are a number of commercially available washes that you can buy for this purpose. This will not work for things on the Dirty Dozen that incorporate the pesticides into their outer skin or the entire fruit. Here is a pesticide wash that you can make yourself. I use this in my kitchen and I highly recommend it. The formula is 1 cup of water, plus one tablespoon of baking soda, plus one cup of apple cider vinegar, plus one half lemon in a sprayer bottle. You should leave the pesticide and antibacterial wash on the produce for about 5 minutes before washing it off. This will also help eliminate any harmful bacteria on the outside of the produce introduced due to picking, storage or transportation.

The 2015 Dirty Dozen list included the following:

- Apples
- Strawberries
- Grapes
- Celery
- Peaches
- Spinach, kale, and collard greens
- Bell peppers: sweet and hot
- Nectarines (imported)
- Cucumbers
- Cherry tomatoes
- Snap peas (imported)
- Potatoes

PFH Action Point

- **Consume a rainbow color of raw fruits and vegetables to obtain the antioxidants we need**
- **Organic is best, but especially those on the Dirty Dozen list from ewg.org**
- **While raw is best, cruciferous veggies can be lightly steamed or sautéed**
- **Decontaminating produce with a wash is desirable, especially if not organic**

When it comes to snacking, nuts and seeds are a good way to go. They are a great source of protein, good fatty acids, and fiber. The only downside to nuts is that they are very calorie dense. It is important to restrain yourself when eating nuts and not consume the whole bag or jar. A handful or a dozen is probably fine. Nuts and seeds should be consumed in their raw form. Roasting and processing nuts and seeds will ruin some of their nutrients. It is best to purchase nuts that are organically grown so that they are free of pesticides and other toxins. This will require some getting used to if you normally consume nuts that are roasted and salted.

Walnuts and almonds have a lot of good research behind them regarding their health benefits. Walnuts have so many good things going for them that they are my choice for the #1 healthy nut to consume. Almonds are probably second place. Cashews, macadamias, and pistachios also have significant health benefits. Sunflower and pumpkin seeds have also been studied and provide numerous health benefits and you will see them on the list of the top iron containing foods.

Nuts and seeds can also be made into butters. Common ones include almond butter and sunflower butter. These make a very nice snack on a piece of celery or other vegetable. Remember, however, they are extremely calorie dense and a little bit adds up to a lot of calories. It should be noted that peanuts are not a nut, but rather a legume. While they do have some nutritional benefits, peanuts are not as healthy as some of the other nuts we have mentioned. As we will see later, peanuts harbor mycotoxins, toxins made by mold. There are numerous mold organisms that can live inside the peanut shell and will contaminate everything the peanuts are put in, including you.

PFH Action Point

- **Nuts and seeds are good snacks, but are very calorie dense**
- **Raw organic are best; avoid roasted, processed nuts and seeds**
- **Walnuts, almonds, macadamias, cashews, pistachios are good**
- **Sunflower, pumpkin seeds are good**
- **Peanuts are a legume, highly contaminated with mycotoxins, and not as healthy**

Let's talk about protein for a moment. In general, Americans eat too much protein. In fact, when you analyze the diets of other cultures, they consume much less protein than we do. Proteins contain amino acids, which are the building blocks of our body. Certain amino acids are termed essential amino acids. Our goal is to consume high quality proteins, whether they are animal or plant based, which will supply all of the essential amino acids. This can become a problem for vegans, but with a little planning and mixing of foods, it is possible. Protein should be consumed at each of our three major meals of the day, but not necessarily for snacks. The amount of protein that's needed is based upon body size, body type, and activity level. For most of us, 15-20 grams of high quality protein at each meal is adequate.

Fish are a great source of protein and good fatty acids. Certain cold water fish, like salmon, are also good sources of omega 3 fatty acids. It is important to note our previous discussions about toxins in the fish, specifically POP's and mercury. Given what we know, I cannot recommend that you eat any freshwater fish. In addition, it is hard to recommend any farm-raised fish as they are often fed GMO foods and are raised in environments where the water is contaminated with toxins. Organically raised fish would be better. The best fish to get are those that are caught wild from the ocean. Again, you must be aware of the fish that contain high levels of mercury and other toxins.

Shrimp can be a great source of protein and good fatty acids. While there has been some misinformation about shrimp and its cholesterol content, I am not very concerned about this. Cholesterol is not a harmful substance. In fact, all of our adrenal hormones are made out of cholesterol. Cholesterol lowering drugs are not fixing our cardiovascular problems. Oxidized LDL cholesterol is a major culprit. However, oxidation occurs due to Free Radicals and this is the real issue that needs to be addressed. Again, shrimp are best obtained wild caught from the ocean or the Gulf instead of farm raised unless you can be sure that they are farm raised in an organic environment. A Consumer Reports article recently detailed the extent of farm-raised shrimp in the US (the vast majority), their countries of origin, and the methods used in their production. I was totally disgusted. I will never eat shrimp from a store or restaurant again without knowing the source. Frying shrimp in unhealthy oils with a breaded coating certainly negates some of the positive health benefits from eating shrimp.

Seafood such as scallops, clams, oysters, and mussels all have the potential to be good sources of protein and good fatty acids. However, these sea animals filter a lot of water through their bodies and may be contaminated with toxins. There is also the issue of how they are raised and harvested and whether they can be contaminated with bacteria. They should never be eaten raw.

PFH Action Point

- **Protein: Americans eat too much of it; 15-20g ok for most people at each meal**
- **Amount at each meal based on size, body type and activity**
- **Fish: be careful of POP's and mercury; no fresh water or farm raised fish-get wild caught from ocean**

- **Shrimp, scallops good if the source is known; wild caught best; no farm raised shrimp**

As we turn our discussion to meat, it is important to emphasize a few points. As we have discussed previously, you must make sure that your meats are free of antibiotics, hormones and GMO feeds. They should be fed an organic diet and be free range, meaning that they are free to roam and eat healthy grasses. Free-range animals are under far less stress than being caged up with hundreds of other animals. All of these precautions will ensure higher nutrient levels and less accumulation of toxins.

Chicken and turkey are very healthy sources of protein and can be very low in bad fats. Generally, their white meat is the best part to eat. Dark meat does contain higher levels of iron, however. In the past, chickens and turkeys were routinely raised with growth hormones, estrogen-like hormones, and antibiotics. It is now much easier to find chicken and turkey free of these toxins. Again, free range and organic is best.

I like a good hamburger or steak on the grill. I know that some of you are probably thinking at this point that I am a vegetarian. While I did spend a year of my life as a vegetarian, doing juicing and totally raw foods, I found that I missed eating meat. I try to be very selective about the red meat that I consume. I certainly don't eat red meat obtained from fast food restaurants. I am not sure what is in it or what toxins it contains. I prefer to buy my own red meat so that I am sure of the source and can cook it the way I desire.

When it comes to beef, grass fed beef is the way to go. The nutritional profile of grass fed beef is much different than grain fed beef. In this country, the vast majority of the red meat that is sold is grain fed. The animals are fed corn, including genetically modified corn, along with other grains to fatten them up. Some may be grass fed for part of their lifetime, but most of their muscle mass is developed eating grains. Grain fed beef is very high in omega 6 fatty acids and not high in the preferred omega 3 fatty acids. This creates more **inflammation**, which is contrary to the lifestyle we are trying to live by. There have been numerous health studies on the negative effects of a diet consisting of large quantities of red meat. However, these studies have not distinguished between grass fed and grain fed beef.

Grass fed beef is the way cows were traditionally raised in this country prior to the last hundred years. Grass fed beef is very high in omega 3 fatty acids. Therefore, it is actually anti-inflammatory and fits in with our new lifestyle. If you prefer to be a vegetarian, I have nothing against that. However, if you prefer to have a good piece of beef occasionally, please try to be selective regarding what type of beef you eat.

The buffalo is a very interesting animal. I love to go to national parks and see a herd of buffalo wandering freely and grazing on grass. They seem to be oblivious to the curious human beings staring at them. They are generally very docile creatures and were a major part of the culture of the American Indians. Our Indians revered the buffalo. They used them for food, clothing, shelter, and other facets of community life. Unfortunately, bison, as they are technically known, were hunted to near extinction in the 1800s.

Bison is making a big comeback. Ranchers have rediscovered the bison and vast herds are reappearing. They are very hearty animals and generally easy to raise. They feed on grasses in the open plains. Bison meat has very little fat and is high in omega 3 fatty acids. It is higher in iron and B12 than beef and has less calories per serving. I love the taste of a bison burger cooked on my grill. It takes a little getting used to eating bison because they are so lean that the steaks and roasts can be a little tough. Using a little creativity in cooking, bison can be a delicious and healthy addition to our **anti-inflammatory lifestyle**.

Another protein to mention is pork. While generally pigs have been looked down upon in western culture, pork can be a healthy addition to our lifestyle. The eating of pigs was prohibited in the Old Testament. In fact, what makes the story of the prodigal son so dramatic is that the prodigal had to work feeding pigs when he ran out of money in the far country. In Jewish culture, there was nothing lower than feeding pigs. In the New Testament, Peter was told to go ahead and eat those animals that had been prohibited in the Old Testament. Therefore, I think it is legitimate to consider eating pork. Obviously, what a pig is fed is critical. Therefore, we need to restrict any pork consumption to organically raised animals only. Hormones and antibiotics are also used to raise nonorganic pigs and so these animals need to be avoided.

Eggs are a great source of protein. While there has been a lot of negative publicity about eggs over the last several decades, due to their cholesterol content, it is clear that eggs do not cause heart or vascular disease. The nutritional content of eggs varies greatly depending on how the chickens are raised and how the eggs are processed. If you do eat eggs, please only eat organic eggs that come from free-range chickens. These will have the highest nutritional content. Beware of eggs produced by nonorganic chickens that are fed hormones and antibiotics. These substances do transfer into the egg.

PFH Action Point

- **Meat should be free range, no antibiotics or hormones, fed an organic diet**
- **Chicken/Turkey: white meat is best, dark meat has more iron**
- **Beef: grain fed high in omega 6 fats (bad), grass fed high in omega 3 fats (better)**
- **Bison is best; it is very low in saturated fat, high in omega 3, and more iron than beef**
- **Pork can be a good source of protein if fed organic foods and no hormones/antibiotics**
- **Eggs are great if organic, free-range**

It is important when preparing protein sources to cook the meat at lower temperatures. Cooking at less than 250 degrees will prevent nitrogen-containing compounds in the meat from converting to a mutagen called benzopyrene. These compounds can induce DNA and RNA mutations and increase the risk of cancer. Thus, on the grill, it might be best to quickly sear the meat at a high temperature for just a moment and then cook at a lower temperature until it is done. This technique also seems to lock in some of the moisture so that the meat is not so dry and tough when it is done.

Related to this discussion of cooking at lower temperatures is the whole subject of Advanced Glycation End Products, or AGE's for short. Besides the production of mutagens, cooking at high temperatures increases the production of AGE's. These are proteins that have been damaged by glycation reactions. These AGE's reflect the accumulation of toxic compounds in the food; the foods with the highest levels of AGE's are also those with the highest levels of mutagens.

The August 2015 issue of Life Extension magazine had a very nice review of the issues involved with AGE's. In summary, when we ingest foods with high levels of AGE's, we increase the glycation of our own proteins and accelerate the aging process. **Inflammation** will result and the risk of cancer goes up substantially. Weight also increases, especially abdominal obesity, due to an AGE called methylglyoxal. Oxidative stress increases as these AGE's take the form of Free Radicals in our bodies.

Since high blood sugar levels also cause protein glycation, Diabetics are especially at risk for significant damage from AGE's. In fact, we can measure this glycation in Diabetics by monitoring their Hemoglobin A1C, a reflection of the amount of glycation done to the Hemoglobin molecule in the last 3 months. This can be correlated to their average blood sugar levels during that time. However, controlling blood sugar is not enough to protect us from the damage caused by AGE's.

When examining the food chart published in the June 2010 issue of the Journal of the American Dietetic Association, it is clear that the foods with the highest AGE's are meats cooked at higher temperatures and highly processed foods. We can protect ourselves, to some degree, by cooking at temperatures less than 300 degrees and not overcooking meats. The highest AGE foods included hot dogs, bacon, sausage, dark meat chicken and turkey, and beef, especially when it is fried or grilled at high heat. Since it is very difficult to avoid ingesting AGE's without going on a totally raw, organic diet, most of us will be exposed to them. Our goal is to minimize our exposure. We will look at some supplements that may be able to protect us from these AGE's later.

PFH Action Point

- **Cook meats at lower temperatures to avoid the production of mutagens and AGE's**
- **Eating foods high in Advanced Glycation End Products (AGE's) will result in damage to our proteins, accelerated aging, cancer, and increased inflammation**
- **Diabetics are at great risk from AGE's as high blood sugars increase glycation and damage**
- **Avoid well done meats, hot dogs, bacon, and highly processed foods.**

Soy is very popular among vegetarians and oriental diets. Soy is a plant protein that is not easily digestible. Fermented soy, such as tempe and miso, are more easily digestible. Beans and lentils are a good source of soy. Remember that in the US, soy is one of the major GMO crops that must be avoided. You can avoid GMO soy by making sure the soy you buy is organic or non-GMO certified. This includes soy products like soy milk, soy lecithin, and soybean oil.

One of the problems with soy is that it is a Phytoestrogen. This means that it binds to estrogen receptors in the body and can increase endometrial and breast cell proliferation. Theoretically, this can result in breast and endometrial cancer. Soy stimulates estrogen receptors, but is weaker than Estradiol and POPs like BPA. Oriental diets that consume a large amount of soy show no increased rates of breast cancer, however.

Consuming a lot of soy affects the conversion of thyroid hormone T4 into T3. We will go into more detail about that later. For now, just know that consuming a large amount of soy can make you feel hypothyroid. I recommend avoiding extracts and supplements like soy isoflavones as they are highly concentrated and will be more potent Phytoestrogens and can affect thyroid hormone conversion even greater.

PFH Action Point

- **Soy can be a good source of protein, but eat it in moderation and make sure it is organic**
- **Tempe and miso are more easily digestible**
- **Soy is a Phytoestrogen, but weaker than Estradiol and BPA**
- **Excess soy consumption affects thyroid hormone conversion**
- **Avoid soy isoflavone supplements**

The subject of fats is very complicated. Over the last several decades, the American public has been fed a lot of misinformation and unfortunately much of this has come from our own government. Studies have been misinterpreted, perhaps intentionally. We now know that not all fat is bad. If we examine the effects of the low fat craze over the past several decades in the United States, it is clear that avoiding fat has not made us healthier. If anything, our health is much worse. We now understand that our brain, nervous system, and certain vitamins need good fats in order to function properly. The question is, what is a good fat?

Let's take a look at some definitions. Omega 6 fatty acids are very prevalent in our food supply. We do need to consume some, but if we get too much omega 6 fatty acids we will increase our **inflammation**. Omega 6's are present in corn, sunflower, cottonseed, safflower, peanut, and soybean oils. If you look at most processed food ingredient labels, you will see these oils. Usually, they show up in cheaper products. They are common in cakes, pies, brownies, cookies, and other treats. They are also commonly used in most chips and other snacks. As covered earlier, omega 6 fatty acids are present in grain fed meats and farm raised fish.

Trans-fatty acids were very commonly used in our food chain until about a decade ago. They are extremely unhealthy and have mostly been eliminated from the food supply. You need to be very vigilant to avoid trans-fatty acids. They show up in cheaper, processed foods and baked goods. They are very inflammatory and need to be avoided in our new lifestyle. Again, omega 6 and trans-fatty acids appear commonly in processed foods, fast foods, fried foods, and sweets.

So what are some of the good fats that we need to consume? Fats are categorized as monounsaturated and polyunsaturated. Monounsaturated fatty acids (MUFA) come from olive, coconut, peanut, canola, sunflower, and sesame oils. They are also present in nuts and seeds. MUFA's are also a component of avocados and olives. MUFA's are a very desirable nutrient to consume in our new **anti-inflammatory lifestyle**. They have been shown in numerous studies to positively impact our health.

Polyunsaturated acids (PUFA) consist of omega 6 and omega 3 fatty acids. We have looked already at omega 6's; now let's take a look at omega 3's. It is generally agreed that we need more omega 3 fatty acids in our diet. However, too much of a good thing is not good. The optimum ratio of omega 6/omega 3 in our diet would be 3 to 1. The average person in the United States consumes a ratio of somewhere between 10-20/1. This shows an overabundance of omega 6 in the diet, which causes **inflammation**. The closer we are to the optimum ratio of 3 to 1, the less **inflammation** we experience. Again, this has important health consequences for our families. Many studies have clearly shown the health benefits of a diet high in omega 3 fatty acids. Since we have no problems obtaining omega 6 in our diet, we must intentionally work at consuming more omega 3 fatty acids.

An omega 3 that is fairly simple and easy to obtain in our diet is alphalinoleic acid (ALA). ALA can be obtained from plants, animals, and beans. Given the right conditions in our body, ALA can be made into the very desirable omega 3's, EPA and DHA. These conditions include having the right vitamins and minerals (B3, B6, C, Zinc, and Magnesium) and not having too high a ratio of omega 6 to omega 3 fatty acids. ALA is present in high amounts in flax, chia, and hemp seeds; it is also present in cauliflower and brussel sprouts. Walnuts are a great source of ALA. Some oils, such as canola and soybean oil, have good concentrations of ALA.

You can obtain EPA and DHA directly in your diet without having to worry about ALA being converted under the right conditions. Good sources of these two omega 3 fatty acids include cold-water ocean fish like salmon, sardines, and cod. Shrimp are also a good source. As we discussed earlier, grass fed meats and free range organic eggs are good sources. While I am not a huge dairy fan, some organic cheese and yogurt can be healthy sources of EPA and DHA while minimizing exposure to harmful environmental toxins. EPA and DHA can also be obtained from supplements; we will look at those later.

Regarding oils, there has been a lot written about the advantages and disadvantages of different oils. I don't want to spend a lot of time going into detail about this because, quite frankly, I don't feel that I am an expert on oils. However, a few generalizations can be made. It is clear from numerous studies that olive oil has numerous health benefits. Any place that you can add some olive oil is a good idea. Hemp and flax oils also have tremendous health benefits. Nut and seed oils, such as walnut, macadamia, and sesame, also are very healthy. Canola and safflower oils are very useful for frying, but remember that canola is mostly GMO in this country unless you buy organic. Oils should be purchased in glass containers and stored in a cool, dry place. Olive oil should be extra virgin, which specifies how it is prepared. Another good preparation method that you may see on organic food labels is expeller pressed. Oils can become rancid and lose their health benefits. So it is important not to use them repeatedly for frying and not to keep them for extended periods of time.

PFH Action Point

- **We need good fats for our brains to work better**
- **Consume less omega 6 and more omega 3 fatty acids to reduce inflammation**

- **Get MUFA's from olives, avocados, and oils like coconut and olive**
- **Omega 3 PUFA's can be obtained from cold water fish and plant sources like hemp, chia and flax**
- **EPA and DHA are desirable omega 3's obtained from foods and supplements**
- **Healthy oils include olive, hemp, flax, and nut oils**

Beans are another great addition to our **anti-inflammatory lifestyle**. Technically, beans are legumes. They are a great source of fiber, protein, ALA, and other nutrients. It is best to buy beans organic, dried, and make them yourself. While this does require a lot of work, the end product will be much healthier and fresher. When cooking beans, it is a good idea to discard the water used to soak the beans in order to decrease potential flatulence. You must remember that canned beans are almost universally lined with BPA to increase their shelf life. An example of a company that does not use BPA in their canned beans is Eden's Organics. A particular mention is deserved for black beans. Black beans are very high in antioxidants, vitamins, and minerals. In general, beans improve digestive health, decrease colon cancer, decrease blood lipids, and decrease blood sugar levels.

Lentils are a very nutritious legume. They are about thirty percent protein, but they are deficient in the amino acids methionine and cysteine. Lentils are very high in fiber. They are also a good source of iron, folate, and vitamin B1. The starch in lentils is very slowly digested, so therefore it is something that diabetics can eat because it will not cause their blood sugar to spike. Lentils are cooked by simmering them in water. Lentils are famous because of the story in the Bible of Jacob and Esau. If you recall, Jacob was making a very tasty lentil stew when Esau came in from hunting and was famished. He sold his birthright for some of Jacob's lentil stew. It must have been very good.

PFH Action Point

- **Beans are a great source of fiber, protein, and ALA; black beans are high in antioxidants**
- **Lentils are a great source of fiber, protein and vitamins; its starch is slowly digested**

Let us examine a few diets from other cultures that are extremely healthy and have proven over time to provide great health benefits. The first is the Mediterranean Diet. This is the traditional dietary pattern of Greece, Southern Italy and Spain. Those cultures have a typical Mediterranean Diet including lots of fresh vegetables and legumes such as beans and lentils. It does not include a lot of sweets and usually fruit is the dessert. The principle source of fats is olive oil, which is used for cooking, salad dressings, and dipping bread. The Mediterranean Diet includes dairy in the form of cheese and yogurt. There is use of unrefined cereals and some bread. The breads are typically whole grain and fairly dense. Fish and poultry are included in small to moderate amounts. Eggs and beef are present in only small amounts. Typically, wine is included with the meal.

When examining the Mediterranean Diet, it seems to meet all of the major criteria that we are discussing for an **anti-inflammatory lifestyle**. There is an emphasis on fresh produce and plant sources of fiber and nutrients. While it does include some dairy, this should be optional. Olive oil supplies the monounsaturated fatty acids (MUFA) and animal protein is kept to a moderate amount. While there is consumption of wheat, the wheat from that area of the world has not been hybridized to produce more gluten as ours has been in America. There is a distinct lack of refined sugars and processed foods. Antioxidants abound in most Mediterranean meals.

Another diet that has proven health benefits is the Oriental Diet. The Oriental Diet is typical in Japan, China, and other countries of Southeast Asia. There is an emphasis on rice and noodles, but these do not contain arsenic in appreciable amounts, as do the same products in

America. The main protein consumed is fish and other seafood. There is a heavy emphasis on fresh vegetables and seaweed. Soup is a frequent dish that is present in the Oriental Diet and is made with vegetables and little meat. There is the consumption of tofu, as we have discussed earlier, without an increase in breast cancers. Sushi is also a part of this diet and does provide significant protein, vitamins, minerals, and good fats. While I am not a sushi fan, I can certainly see potential benefits in consuming it.

The Oriental Diet does not typically contain cow's milk or beef. A lot has been made of this in studies such as "The China Study." The premise is that the lack of cow's milk and beef in the Chinese Diet has contributed to their overall better health and longevity. While the Oriental Diet clearly does not contain cow's milk or beef in appreciable quantities, it is hard to draw the conclusion that cow's milk or beef are responsible for all of our ailments in the United States. We will be examining cow's milk later, but for now I have to agree that there is little place for it in our diet. While we can live very nicely without eating beef, given the right precautions, beef can be a very healthy addition to our diet without creating excess **inflammation.**

PFH Action Point

- **The Mediterranean Diet has been well studied for its health benefits**
- **The Oriental Diet is also very healthy and deserves your attention**
- **Both diets stress raw fruits and vegetables, small amounts of high quality animal protein, legumes, some healthy grains, good fats and little processed foods and sugar**

As we examine the diets of other cultures in the world, we can see that there are numerous healthy foods available in other countries that we do not have access to here in America. Some of these are highly nutritious and have earned the term "super foods." I have spent a lot of time researching "super foods" for my patients. Typically, they can be combined together in a highly nutritious drink, a smoothie. I have one of these super food smoothies most mornings to start my day. Let's take a look at some of these "super foods" and how we can combine them together to aid in our **anti-inflammatory lifestyle**.

Super food smoothies are part of a raw, living, whole foods diet. The ingredients are not processed or heated as this will destroy some of the nutrients. The nutrients will be available in an easily digestible and absorbable form. This is of great benefit for those with intestinal problems and malabsorption issues. This includes those with irritable bowel syndrome, leaky gut syndrome, and inflammatory bowel disease.

Our super foods will be coming mostly from other countries. They are not readily available here in the United States. You cannot walk into a typical grocery store and find most of this. However, you can obtain these super foods on the internet, in health food stores, and in certain progressive grocery stores and warehouses. Super foods are very nutrient dense and have been used in other cultures for thousands of years. They have lots of science and research behind them. It should be stressed that you must buy super foods in their organic form due to the risk of pesticides, some of which may be used in other countries, but are banned here in the United States because of their toxicity. Using reputable companies, such as Navitas Naturals and Nutiva, will ensure the quality of these organic super foods.

One of the most important ingredients in our super food smoothie will be the protein that we are using. I have issues with a lot of powdered proteins including whey, soy, and rice. After much research, I have come to the conclusion that the optimal protein for our super food smoothie is hemp. Yes, I said hemp. Hemp seeds are harvested from the cannabis plant. While this is the same plant that is grown to produce marijuana, it is a totally different variety. There are over 20 varieties of cannabis plants. This particular variety has minimal THC. What makes hemp protein so noteworthy is that it is one of the few complete plant proteins. That means that it has all of the essential amino acids that are needed by the human body. Hemp is very high in omega 6 fatty acids (GLA) and omega 3's (SDA) in a 3 to 1 ratio. This is the optimum omega 6 to omega 3 ratio and is highly valued in diets and very difficult to find. Hemp is very high in fiber, chlorophyll, and other important nutrients.

The history of hemp is very interesting. Hemp was an important part of the diet and commerce of the American colonies. Thomas Jefferson and George Washington were hemp farmers. Because of the breeding of cannabis plants to produce more THC, hemp farming was eventually banned in the United States. Today, most of our hemp protein is imported from South America and Canada. It is a shame that this very important and profitable commodity is not being grown in our country. As with other super foods, hemp should be obtained in its organic form. It can be purchased in seeds, powder, and oil. It can be added to salads, smoothies, and various recipes. I have found that hemp powder is the most convenient form for our super food smoothies.

Another important super food is chia. Chia seeds were a staple of the Aztecs, Mayans, and Inca Indians. They have been used for thousands of years. It is reported that runners would carry pouches of chia seeds with them in order to replenish their energy on their journeys. Chia seeds are very high in omega 3 fatty acids, protein, fiber, and other nutrients. Chia seeds can be soaked, sprouted, and ground into a powder. When using chia seeds in our super food smoothies, it is best to add them to some liquid and let them soak for 5 to 10 minutes. They then form a nutritious gel that is much easier to work with and will be more easily absorbed.

Another important super food is flax. Flax seeds are talked about a lot in nutritional circles these days and have even found their way into mainstream food stores. Flax seeds are very high in omega 3 fatty acids, fiber and protein. They are also high in a substance called lignans. These lignans in flax may protect against cardiovascular disease and certain cancers such as breast cancer. Flax seeds can be ground into a powder, which will be easier to use in our super food smoothies. Again, obtaining flax in the organic form is desirable.

Cacao is the Indian name for the cocoa bean. Cocoa beans are actually a vegetable. We will be examining cocoa a little bit later as we look at antioxidant foods. Cocoa is the highest antioxidant food in the world. Per gram of cocoa, there are more important and helpful antioxidants than in any other food. Cocoa can be made into a butter or paste and ground into a powder. As we will be discussing later, it is important to obtain cocoa in a cold processed form that preserves its nutrients. Once cocoa is heated over 110 degrees, it loses many of its antioxidants and healthy enzymes. Finding this cold processed cocoa is a little bit difficult. A good source is a company called Navitas Naturals, which you can find on the internet.

Our super food smoothies will also need to have some fruits in them. One of the highest antioxidant fruits in the world is the Acai berry. Acai is a fascinating fruit. It is from the Amazon rainforest. It is very high in omega 3 fatty acids, vitamins, and minerals. Acai berries have arrived at many grocery stores in the form of a juice, either on its own or combined with other fruits. Juice is not the preferred way to use this super food. The sugar content is enormous. If it has been pasteurized or otherwise processed, it has lost a lot of its antioxidant benefits. It is best to obtain Acai as a freeze-dried powder to add to our super food smoothie.

Other super food fruits that we can use for our smoothies include Maqui berries, Goji berries, Mulberries, Goldenberries, and Blueberries. These are also very healthy to snack on, either raw or dried. Since Blueberries are very highly contaminated with pesticides, it is essential to obtain them in the organic form. All of these berries are very high in different kinds of antioxidants, so it is a good idea to mix them.

Another super food fruit is the Pomegranate. The Pomegranate is an ancient super fruit from the Bible and is well known throughout the Middle Eastern cultures. The Pomegranate is very high in antioxidants, fiber, vitamins, and minerals. Most of the nutrition is in the Pomegranate seeds. The seeds can be eaten raw or they can be freeze-dried and ground into a powder. It is this pomegranate powder that will be a helpful addition to our super food smoothies.

Maca is a root grown in the Andes Mountains in South America. It has been a staple of the Indians living in those areas for thousands of years. Maca is very high in nutrients and fiber. Of interest is the fact that

Maca is an adaptagen that assists the adrenal glands to adapt to stress. Maca root can be ground into a powder that is very easy to use in our smoothies.

Another interesting super food is Wheatgrass. While you may be thinking that wheatgrass has wheat in it, this is not the case. Wheatgrass is very high in vitamins and nutrients. It also contains chlorophyll, which is the green pigment in plants and is very healthy for us to ingest. Wheatgrass is a natural detoxifying agent. While you can obtain wheatgrass in its natural form, which is a grass, and add it to your smoothie, it is also available in a freeze-dried powder. The powder is much more concentrated and a little easier to use in our smoothies.

Another super food, which is well known to us, is Coconut. Coconut is a monounsaturated fatty acid (MUFA) with numerous health benefits. We have already identified coconut oil as a great source of good fatty acids. It is also fairly easy to cook with. Coconut can be made into flour that can be used as a substitute for wheat in numerous recipes. Coconut is good to just snack on raw. For our super food smoothie, we will be using coconut milk. The newest craze seems to be coconut water. Coconut water does contain electrolytes and other nutrients and is certainly a better rehydrating agent that using commercially available electrolyte drinks that contain high fructose corn syrup, bromine, and other toxins.

My patients often ask me where they can obtain the ingredients to make our super food smoothies. I have found two companies to be particularly good sources of organic ingredients at a reasonable cost. One is Navitas Naturals and the other is Nutiva. Both can be obtained directly from their websites, but they are also available on both Amazon and Swanson. There are probably other good sources for our ingredients as well. These are just two companies that I have investigated more thoroughly.

Here is an example of a super food smoothie that I use most mornings. It is a little complicated so you can start off with something a little simpler if you want.

SUPER FOOD SMOOTHIE

½ cup Coconut milk

½ cup George's Aloe Vera Liquid

4 tbsp Nutiva High Fiber Hemp Protein Powder

1 tbsp Organic Flax Powder

1 tbsp Organic Chia Seeds (Soak for 5 to 10 minutes)

2-3 tbsp Navitas Cacoa Powder

1 tbsp Navitas Maca Powder

1 tsp Navitas Superfruit Blend

1 tbsp Organic Wheatgrass Powder

½ banana + ½ cup frozen organic blueberries

Add Stevia or organic cane sugar to taste

This amazing super food smoothie contains approximately 16 ounces of the highest quality nutrients you can put into your body. What a great way to start your day! This smoothie contains 27 grams of vegetable protein in a very absorbable form. It contains 36 grams of fiber. Given that we need to be consuming over 35 grams of fiber per day, you will already be getting it at breakfast. This smoothie contains 9600 milligrams of plant based omega 3 fatty acids, which, as we discussed previously, will be converted to DHA and EPA in your body given the right conditions. Our smoothie contains 455 calories if you are using Stevia to sweeten it. If you are trying to restrict your caloric intake, then you may want to cut back on some of the fruit.

I highly recommend you consider adding super food smoothies to your **anti-inflammatory lifestyle**. You can use them as a meal substitute any time of the day. You can also create many other healthy smoothies. There are many recipes online and I refer you to the Navitas Naturals website for a more thorough discussion and those recipes.

PFH Action Point

- Super food Smoothies are a great way to supercharge your body with nutrients
- They can serve as a meal replacement, as long as they have adequate protein
- Use only organic sources for your super foods
- They will supply antioxidants, strengthen your immune system, and aid in detoxification

Chapter 8
Don't Live to Eat!

In our last chapter, we looked at the cornerstone of our treatment pyramid, which is nutrition. We were able to identify things that you can do nutritionally to support our **anti-inflammatory lifestyle**. We decided that it was better to eat for a purpose, which is to supply our body with the building blocks and nutrients it needs for repair and a healthy immune system. It is better to eat to live than to live to eat.

In this chapter, we will be looking at the things that we have been doing as a culture that are creating **inflammation** and the diseases that we are seeing reach epidemic proportions in our country. While some of these things may make us feel better for a time, and even taste good at the moment, we need to take a more long-term view of their effects on our bodies. Again, we must acknowledge the fact that what we have been doing has not worked very well and we need to change now.

Probably the number one thing on my list of things that we must change, because of its negative health effect, is the consumption of wheat. While we have been taught for many decades in this nation that wheat is good for us, it is clear now that is not the case. Just ask anyone on a gluten free or wheat free diet how they feel now compared to how they were when they were eating wheat. They will tell you that they feel so much better since they have eliminated wheat from their diet. I can share with you numerous patient examples from my practice of people who felt horrible and consistently tested negative for wheat allergy. However, once they eliminated wheat from their diet, their health turned around dramatically. While this may not be true in every person's life, wheat is certainly one of the contributing factors to our national **inflammation** epidemic.

So why is wheat so bad for us? After all, wheat has been consumed in many cultures for thousands of years. It is important to understand that the wheat we are consuming in America is no longer the grain mentioned in the Bible. The major harvests that are mentioned in the Bible for ancient Israel are the wheat and the barley harvests. Much of community life revolved around harvesting these very important and nutritious grains. In a culture where there is little consumption of processed foods, sugar, and other bad carbohydrates, the consumption of wheat could be acceptable. Well, that is certainly not the situation in our country.

Wheat in the United States has been hybridized numerous times to increase yield, increase gluten content, and to resist disease. While some consider this to be genetic modification, it is not the same as what is done with GMO foods. We will be looking at GMO foods shortly. This simply involves the manipulation of strains and crossbreeding for a desired effect. Hybridization has been done with many other plants throughout the centuries. In this case, hybridization has resulted in wheat becoming one of the highest glycemic foods in our diet.

As a result of the increased gluten content of United States wheat, gluten allergy (Celiac Disease) and gluten sensitivities are very common in our population. Celiac Disease is the result of **inflammation** of the lining of the intestinal tract. While published studies have shown a very small percentage of people have Celiac disease and true gluten allergy, the number of people is rising rapidly. Of more concern to me are the number of people that have gluten sensitivity. The standardized testing that we do for gluten allergy is negative in these patients. The only real way to detect gluten sensitivity is to eliminate wheat and gluten from your diet for several months and see how you feel. Some of the symptoms of gluten sensitivity include Irritable Bowel Syndrome, Leaky Gut Syndrome, malabsorption, diarrhea, weight gain, fatigue, skin rashes and itching, headaches, and a host of other symptoms.

So what is gluten? Gluten is one of the proteins that is found in wheat. In fact there are over twenty proteins found in wheat. Gliadin is another protein that is commonly tested in panels looking for Celiac Disease. Gluten is also found in oats, rye, barley, and spelt. Unless a grain specifically has a statement on the packaging declaring that it is certified gluten free, it is common that it is produced in a plant where gluten is also processed and may have contaminated that grain. While this tiny amount of gluten may not be of concern for most of us, for those with Celiac Disease it can be debilitating. Gluten helps to increase the shelf life of wheat products and so therefore increases profitability. Gluten also makes it easier to bake with wheat ingredients.

The result of the hybridization of wheat, as mentioned, has been a very high glycemic food. The Glycemic Index is a measurement that enables us to compare foods regarding their ability to stimulate the Pancreas to secrete insulin. It is this insulin secretion that stresses our bodies and causes us to turn sugar into fat. Constant stimulation of our pancreas with high glycemic foods can result in diabetes. The Glycemic Index of whole grain bread is higher than sucrose. Sucrose is sugar. In fact, two slices of whole wheat bread has a higher glycemic index than a can of regular soda or a candy bar! Think about this. What we have been told to eat for decades in our country as a healthy breakfast, which is two slices of whole wheat bread with a glass of orange juice, is worse for our body than having a can of soda and a candy bar for breakfast.

Another interesting aspect of wheat is that it increases production of a hormone called Grehlin. Grehlin is one of the hormones that tell our body that we are hungry and we need to eat. Therefore, eating wheat results in us wanting to eat more. Wheat also decreases the production of Leptin. Leptin is a hormone that tells our body to burn fat. Therefore, wheat causes us to store fat. Next time you are tempted to have that big sub sandwich, or that big bowl of pasta, remember that the wheat will increase Grehlin production and cause you to want to eat more; the wheat will increase insulin secretion and will result in the conversion of sugar into fat; and the wheat will suppress Leptin production so that you will store all the sugar as fat, usually around your waist.

Wheat is also an exogenous endorphin. An endorphin is a feel good hormone. In many ways, naturally produced endorphins in our body act like a narcotic. Wheat can actually give us a "high" and create a cycle of addiction whereby we want to eat more wheat. In addition, dopamine is stimulated in the brain when wheat is consumed. This creates a brain reward pathway that is similar to other addictions. This is why patients often describe to me a feeling that they "crave" bread and pasta. Wheat truly behaves as an addicting substance.

The consumption of wheat increases visceral fat. This is the fat that lines our internal organs and is not visible externally. You can look fairly thin and still carry around a lot of excess visceral fat. This fat results in **inflammation**, insulin resistance and hormone imbalance. As we have discussed previously, blood sugar spikes caused by the consumption of wheat are very stressful on the pancreas and your adrenal glands.

The consumption of wheat also causes the production of Advanced Glycation End Products (AGE), more so than many other sugars. An example of an AGE that we measure commonly in medicine is the Hemoglobin A1C. While this is commonly felt to be a reflection of the average blood sugar over the past three months, it is really a measure of the production of AGE's over the past three months. AGE's result in accelerated aging, as well as Coronary Artery Disease, Cardiovascular Disease, Peripheral Vascular Disease, Kidney disease, dementia, arthritis, and skin aging. As you can see, these AGE's are correlated with many of the chronic diseases we are dealing with in our country and are related to sugar intake.

An excellent reference on the subject of wheat is a book by William Davis, M.D. and entitled <u>Wheat Belly</u>. I encourage you to examine this book if you are interested in learning more about the negative health consequences of a diet consuming wheat.

PFH Action Point

- **Wheat is a high glycemic food with many negative health consequences**

- **Gluten allergy (Celiac Disease) is not common, but gluten sensitivity is**
- **Wheat produces hormonal changes that cause you to eat more and store sugar as fat, especially around your waist and internal organs**
- **Wheat produces addiction-like changes in the brain, making it hard to quit**
- **Production of AGE's increase chronic disease and premature aging**

Another change that we must make is to reduce our sugar intake. The average American consumes 152 pounds of sugar per year, or three pounds per week! This has been steadily increasing over the last century. Sugar goes by a lot of names. These include glucose, sucrose, maltose, dextrose, lactose, sorbitol, High Fructose Corn Syrup (HFCS), corn syrup, fruit juice concentrate, honey, and molasses. While all of these sugars may differ by their chemical structure and by taste, they all produce the same response in the body. They are still sugar. It should be noted that products that are termed "gluten free" and "low fat" often have a lot of sugar in order to make them taste better. Americans definitely have a sweet tooth.

Sugar, by whatever name it goes by, causes insulin secretion. This results in increased stress on our pancreas and causes the storage of sugar as fat. Over time, this pancreatic stress and constant need for insulin will result in insulin resistance. This means that the insulin becomes less and less effective at doing its job. The result is an elevated blood sugar and the need to secrete more insulin. Over time, the pancreas will lose its ability to keep up with the blood sugar demands and the result is Diabetes Mellitus. This is commonly called Type II Diabetes. If the production of insulin should decline to levels that no longer meet body sugar demands, this is termed Type I Diabetes. There is a lot of overlap between the two types.

Another issue related to sugar consumption is high fructose corn syrup (HFCS). We will be examining HFCS shortly. In addition, there is the issue of genetically modified sugar from sugar beets that is used extensively in our country, especially in processed foods.

We have been taught for decades that it is a good thing to have a glass of orange juice in the morning with your breakfast. Did you know that 12 ounces of orange juice has nine teaspoons of sugar? Yes, there are other vitamins and nutrients that may be in the orange juice that are beneficial for us, but the concentrated fructose in the orange juice is equivalent to nine teaspoons of sugar. If you think about that, there is the same amount of sugar in a can of regular soda. So, would it be ok to have a can of soda with your breakfast? While many people do that, it is certainly not a healthy idea.

Instead of using sugar to sweeten things such as coffee, tea, or our super food smoothies, try using alternative sweeteners. Remember that all of the artificial sweeteners are toxins. However, Stevia is perfectly safe. Stevia is made from the leaves of a plant that has a natural sweetness without affecting significantly the secretion of insulin. It would be best to use organic Stevia. Other alternatives include Agave Nectar, Palm sugar, and Coconut sugar. Remember that these other sugars do stimulate the secretion of insulin from your pancreas, but not to the extent as sucrose and fructose.

PFH Action Point

- **Americans eat 3 pounds of sugar per week**
- **Sugar goes by many names, but it is still sugar; High Fructose Corn Syrup is the worst**
- **Excess sugar intake results in diabetes and many health problems**
- **Juice contains large amounts of fructose, a potent sugar and potential toxin**
- **Use Stevia to sweeten drinks and foods**

An interesting discussion related to the topic of sugar intake concerns brain health. There has been a lot of research in recent years concerning the relationship between diet and the health of our brains. Can nutrition affect the development of dementia and other neurological disorders? A good review of this topic has been published by David Perlmutter, M.D. in his book, <u>Grain Brain</u>. I highly recommend that you read it.

It is clear from the research that sugar is a toxin and causes dementia. The Mayo Clinic published a study in January of 2012 and concluded that there was an 89% increase in dementia when using a high carbohydrate diet and a 44% decrease in dementia when using a high fat diet. This flies in the face of most of the nutritional information that we have been taught over the past fifty years. I was always taught that the brain needed sugar to burn as fuel in order to function properly and that fat poisoned the brain. This could not be further from the truth. Apparently the brain prefers healthy fats to burn as fuel to protein and sugars. Sugar is actually detrimental to our brain function.

The higher our carbohydrate intake is, the worse our brain functions. This is due to decreased mitochondrial function among other things. The mitochondria are the little energy producing factories within our cells. The more sugar we ingest, the worse our mitochondrial function and the production of needed energy for our brains. Increased sugar intake also causes **inflammation** and Free Radical production. We have looked at Free Radicals and their effect on our bodies in a previous chapter. Since we are trying to have an **anti-inflammatory lifestyle**, it is clear that a high carbohydrate diet is not consistent with that.

Those who specialize in the care of children with ADHD have known for a long time that taking these children off of sugar and gluten will greatly improve their symptoms. They discovered a long time ago that good fats in their diet and giving them vitamin D3 supplements also improved their cognitive function. Since heavy metal toxicity can also play a role in ADHD, detoxification of these children should be undertaken before prescribing amphetamines for their condition.

Studies in the New England Journal of Medicine and the Journal of the American Medical Association have uniformly shown that a high fat diet wins over a high carbohydrate diet in nearly every cardiovascular risk parameter. That means the more good fats that you consume, and the less sugar that you consume, the less chance that you will develop cardiovascular disease. Again, this seems contrary to everything that we have been taught for the past fifty years. We have been taught that fat and cholesterol are not good for the heart and therefore our nation embarked on this low fat diet campaign that clearly has not helped us to be healthier. It certainly has enabled pharmaceutical companies to convince generations of doctors to prescribe cholesterol-lowering drugs and they have profited greatly from this.

We have all seen the food pyramid of 1992 and children have been taught that in schools now for over 20 years. In the food pyramid, the USDA tells us what to eat to have a longer and healthier life. The bottom of the food pyramid (what we need to eat more) includes grains and fruits. The top of the food pyramid (what we need to avoid) includes fats. We now can see that this is the exact opposite of what we should be doing. It seems to me that there was a conflict of interest here. The USDA represents the food growers and producers in our country. Since the introduction of the food pyramid, diabetes has tripled and other chronic diseases have steadily increased. It is obvious that the food pyramid needs to be totally overhauled.

As we consider the whole subject of brain health, it is clear that the brain will use anything for fuel, but it functions more efficiently by burning fats. There is much less production of Free Radicals when the brain has fat to use for fuel versus sugars. With fat as a fuel, the brain actually undergoes Mitochondrial Biogenesis, which is the growth of new mitochondria. This is obviously very beneficial for the function of our brains as it creates more energy for brain functions. There is also an increase in BNF (Brain-Derived Neurotropic Factor) and the increased growth of neurons (brain cells). With fats as fuel, there is increased neuroplasticity, which is the increase in neural connections resulting in increased memory, focus, and reaction times. There is also increased repair of damaged neurons.

So if fats are the best fuel for our brain to work the most efficiently and be as healthy as possible, what are the best choices in fats for us to eat as part of our **anti-inflammatory lifestyle**? Also we need to be concerned about bad fats producing lipophyllic toxins as they are burned for fuel. These toxins generate Free Radicals. In addition, the fats we consume may already contain toxins, such as Endocrine Disruptors, that will contribute to Free Radical production as they are burned for fuel. The best good fat choices seem to be organic olive oil, organic butter, organic free-range eggs, and grass fed free-range meats. Super foods we have discussed, like hemp, chia, and flax, are good sources of healthy fats. Nuts and nut oils can provide our brains with healthy fats.

PFH Action Point

- **Sugar is a toxin to our brain and you must reduce sugar consumption**
- **Your brain needs good fats to work most efficiently: organic olive oil, organic butter, organic free-range eggs, and grass fed free-range meats; super foods like hemp, chia, and flax; and nuts and nut oils**
- **High carbohydrate diets result in Free Radical production, poor brain health, and many chronic diseases**
- **The USDA Food Pyramid needs to be overhauled as it stresses eating the wrong things**

What is the truth about fructose? There is a lot of conflicting information in the media about fructose and High Fructose Corn Syrup (HFCS). On the one side, scientists and nutritionists who have studied fructose and High Fructose Corn Syrup tell us that they are toxins. On the other side, other scientists supported by the food industry are telling us that they are just another sugar and perfectly healthy for our bodies. Who do we believe?

After researching fructose and High Fructose Corn Syrup for some time, I am convinced that fructose is a bad sugar, but High Fructose Corn Syrup is a toxin. Just like all of the simple sugars that we have examined, it is clearly best to reduce the consumption of fructose in general. However, given the effects of HFCS on our bodies, we need to avoid it totally. With wheat, HFCS is largely responsible for the obesity epidemic in America. It is in everything; especially beverages like sodas, sports drinks, fruit juices, sweet teas, and processed foods. I am always amazed that you can find HFCS in things like barbecue sauce and ketchup. Since it is hidden in so many things, it is very important to read labels and to recognize it. It may just be called corn syrup nowadays.

Robert Lustig, M.D, did a wonderful review of the whole HFCS controversy. This video can be seen on YouTube and is entitled "Sugar: The Bitter Truth." I found this video to be extremely informative. In fact, I took notes during the entire presentation. I would definitely encourage anyone interested in an **anti-inflammatory lifestyle** to view this video.

Fructose is metabolized in our liver directly to fat. This is not what happens to sugars like sucrose and dextrose. In fact, this fructose metabolism by the liver looks exactly like how alcohol is metabolized by the liver. Thus, as far as our body is concerned, the consumption of one can of regular soda is equivalent to drinking one can of beer. All of the same effects and complications that occur with alcohol use can occur with fructose consumption.

When examining the metabolism of fructose, studies have shown that consuming one can of soda per day will result in the average person gaining 15.5 pounds of fat per year! This is very concerning as most people are drinking more than one can of soda per day, especially our young people. Is it any wonder then that we have an obesity epidemic, given the love affair we have with sugar sweetened beverages in our society?

For many years, we have been told it is a good idea to feed our children fruit juice. In fact, it is a standard part of breakfast and lunch programs, especially in the inner cities. What does all this fruit juice consumption do to our children? It has resulted in poor cognitive function, lower test results, and more behavioral problems. Yet we are still doing it. We are serving the fruit juice to children in juice boxes that contain plastics and other toxins. It may not be 100% juice and may also be sweetened with HFCS and/or other sugars. This is not the way to create future generations of Americans with good brain function. It is best to eat the whole piece of fruit and not the concentrated juice. The pulp of the fruit actually decreases the absorption of the fructose.

HFCS causes Non-Alcoholic Fatty Liver (NAFL), which is dramatically increasing in our nation. It should be easier for us to understand why this is happening now. The HFCS is metabolized just like alcohol and so it produces the same side effects and complications. Just like alcohol abuse causes cirrhosis, so HFCS abuse causes NAFL. HFCS also increases triglyceride levels and small, dense LDL cholesterol. This causes atherosclerosis and heart disease. Remember, it is not the cholesterol that is the problem, but the triglycerides and this oxidized small, dense LDL cholesterol. That is why countless billions of prescriptions for statin drugs have not fixed our vascular problems in this country.

HFCS is made from GMO corn. We will discuss GMO foods later. It is also one of the most mercury-contaminated food ingredients because of the way it is made. HFCS causes an increase in visceral fat, which results in increased **inflammation**, insulin resistance, diabetes, and hormone imbalances. If we are going to embark upon an **anti-inflammatory lifestyle**, we must eliminate all HFCS from our diet. We also must stop consuming fruit juice.

PFH Action Point

- **High Fructose Corn Syrup (HFCS) is a toxin and is in a lot of foods and drinks**
- **HFCS is largely responsible, with wheat, for our obesity epidemic; drink 1 can of soda per day and you will gain 15.5 lbs of fat per year**

- **Fructose is metabolized in the liver to fat, just like alcohol, and causes Non-Alcoholic Fatty Liver (NAFL)**
- **Fruit juice should be avoided; eat the whole piece of fruit instead**
- **HFCS is made from GMO corn and is contaminated with mercury; it increases insulin resistance and diabetes**

Another thing that we need to limit in our **anti-inflammatory lifestyle** is the consumption of dairy. Again, this will not be easy. I actually do like some hard cheeses and some organic ice cream. However, many people are allergic to cow's milk and to its components. Cow's milk is for cows; it is not for human beings. In fact, all mention of milk in the Bible concerns goat's milk. Goat's milk has a much different structure than cow's milk and is much less allergenic. It would be okay to have some organic goat's milk or goat's milk cheese occasionally.

Remember that toxins such as hormones, antibiotics, POPs and other Endocrine Disruptors are frequently found in milk. Some of this is reduced when you use organic products. Dairy includes soft cheeses, yogurt, ice cream, and sour cream. Hard cheeses have less milk in them, but people can still react to them. It is best to limit your consumption of cow's milk dairy. If you are lactose intolerant, or have Irritable Bowel Syndrome (IBS) or Leaky Gut Syndrome, you need to avoid it totally.

PFH Action Point
- **Avoid cow's milk and milk products**
- **Goat's milk and products may be safer**
- **If you do have some dairy, limit the amount and use organic products**
- **Avoid cow's milk dairy if you react to it, have Leaky Gut or IBS**

We mentioned artificial sweeteners briefly, but I want to spend more time on this subject. The most common artificial sweeteners used in our country are aspartame (Nutrasweet), saccharin (Sweet and Low), and sucralose (Splenda). Not only do they appear in diet drinks and foods, but in many products that are labeled "low sugar" or "reduced sugar" or "low calorie." After studying these substances, it is clear that we have replaced sugar with toxins. How these artificial sweeteners were released into the American food chain is a mystery to me.

The research done on the health effects of Aspartame has been extensive and well documented. Adverse effects include brain excitation (ADHD and seizures), headaches, depression, anxiety, memory loss, sleep disorders and brain damage. Saccharin is a known carcinogen in laboratory animals and has no business being consumed by human beings. Research is quickly emerging about the health effects of Sucralose, especially how it relates to our gut function. Anyone who has ever had loose stools after consuming Sucralose can attest to this.

Let us focus for a little bit on diet sodas and their negative health effects. A study done by the University of Texas showed that consuming one diet soda per day would result in a 70% increase in waist circumference in one year. This is very concerning. However, even worse was the fact that consuming two or more diet sodas a day resulted in a 500% increase in waist circumference in a year. Given the fact that many people are consuming 4 to 6 or more diet sodas a day, is it any wonder that we have an obesity epidemic? We were told that consuming diet soda was better for us because we would be consuming less sugar and have less diabetes. That has certainly not turned out to be the case.

A Danish study showed that consuming 1 to 3 diet sodas per day resulted in a 38% increase in preterm births. Consuming 4 or more diet sodas per day resulted in a 78% increase in preterm births. This is extremely concerning given the escalating rate of miscarriages that are seen in developed countries around the world. Could it be related to diet soda consumption?

A study in the Journal of General Internal Medicine from January 30, 2012 revealed that consuming 1 diet soda per day increased the risk of heart attack, stroke, and vascular events by 43%. Again, is it any wonder that we still have an incredibly high rate of heart and vascular disease in our country? A Harvard study showed a 30% decrease in kidney function in women that consumed 2 or more diet sodas per day. The United States already has one of the highest rates of kidney disease in the world. Could our consumption of diet sodas be contributing to that?

After looking at all of the data, it is clear that diet soda is a poison and must be eliminated from your life. If you are addicted to diet sodas and are consuming more than four per day on a regular basis, you will probably need to slowly decrease your consumption. Otherwise, you may go into withdrawal, either from the lack of caffeine or from the lack of these artificial sweeteners. It is better to replace the caffeine with some coffee or green tea and then slowly cut back on that.

PFH Action Point

- **Artificial sweeteners replace sugar with toxins that negatively impact our health**
- **Aspartame causes brain excitation, headaches, mood and sleep disorders**
- **Diet sodas cause obesity, preterm births, vascular and kidney disease**
- **Diet soda is a poison and must be eliminated from your life**

I want to take some time to closely examine the controversy regarding GMO (genetically modified organism) foods. I tried to enter into this study of GMO foods with an open mind. However, something inside me told me that it just seemed wrong to start changing the genetic structure of God's creation. By altering this genetic structure of our crops, would we be creating a monster that would quickly get out of control and destroy us? While this sounds like science fiction perhaps, I do not believe that it is. GMO foods have generated organizations, ballot initiatives, and the spending of untold millions of dollars by large agricultural and chemical companies to better inform the public. GMO labeling initiatives in numerous states have been vigorously opposed by large corporations. If GMO foods are safe for us, why would there be so much opposition to require labeling of products containing GMO foods?

GMO foods actually involve genetic engineering. Unlike the hybridization of wheat, the genetic structure of the GMO food has been altered to make it disease or pest resistant, increase its yield, or to make it herbicide or pesticide resistant. An example is Round Up Ready Corn by Monsanto. Here corn has been genetically engineered to resist damage by the herbicide Round Up (glyphosate). Foods may also be altered genetically to incorporate a pesticide into its structure in order to control pests that may attack that plant. Some of these pesticides actually cause the bug's stomach to explode after they ingest it. What does consumption of this GMO food, containing this pesticide gene, do to our guts?

It is clear from studies that GMO foods do not behave as the real food, but generate an immune response such as by a foreign invader. The result is **inflammation** and disease. In fact, animals fed GMO feeds can get sick and die more frequently than animals not fed those products.

In the United States, GMO foods include over 90% of the corn crop and will therefore appear in corn flower, corn oil syrup, corn starch and High Fructose Corn Syrup (HFCS). Over 90% of the soybean crop in the United States is GMO and will affect soy protein, soy milk, soybean oil, soy flour, and tofu. Other significant GMO crops and products include cottonseed oil, canola oil, vegetable oil, maltodextrin, yellow squash, zucchini, Hawaiian papaya, and sugar from sugar beets. As you can see, GMO foods will show up in a large amount of the products that you buy at the grocery store if you are not careful. In addition, GMO foods are commonly fed to our livestock in their grain.

So what are we to do to avoid GMO foods as part of our **anti-inflammatory lifestyle**? After all, there must be a reason that the European Union has banned all imports of Monsanto GMO corn due to their animal studies showing the development of cancer and sickness. Only buy products that are certified organic. Another acceptable alternative is to use products that say "Non-GMO Project Verified." This is especially important for any of the products listed above that have a high percentage of GMO contamination. You can get an app from the Institute for Responsible Technology that will help you know which foods are GMO risks.

The FDA refuses to make labeling of our foods for GMO ingredients mandatory. Why? Monsanto and DuPont are pouring millions of dollars into opposing state labeling ballot initiatives. Why? Don't we have a right to know what we are eating? Go to the Institute for Responsible Technology website to learn more and get involved.

PFH Action Point

- **GMO foods have been genetically altered to resist disease, pests, herbicides or pesticides**
- **They can generate an immune response, increase inflammation, and increase your risk of diseases**
- **Includes most corn, soy, canola oil, cottonseed oil, vegetable oil, maltodextrin, yellow squash, zucchini, Hawaiian papaya, and sugar from sugar beets**
- **Avoid GMO foods by buying organic or "Non-GMO Project Verified"**

It is important in our **anti-inflammatory lifestyle** to eat more organic produce. This is certainly essential for produce on the list called the "Dirty Dozen." These are the fruits and vegetables that have the highest level of pesticide contamination in our nation. In many cases, it is impossible to get the pesticides totally off of these fruits and vegetables. By eating organic produce, there is much less chance of pesticide contamination. In addition, organic produce has been shown to have 25% higher nutrient levels in several studies. Produce on the "Clean Fifteen" have less pesticide contamination and theoretically could be consumed in a non-organic form. You can get these lists and apps for your phone from Environmental Working Group. I highly recommend switching totally to organic produce when possible and finances permit it.

Organic products avoid all GMO ingredients. This removes the possibility of consuming GMO foods from your new lifestyle. Organic meats also avoid the use of growth hormones and routine antibiotics. Buying organic produce also helps small farmers. For packaged foods, buying organic avoids many harmful additives, chemicals, and preservatives. However, it does not eliminate wheat from the ingredient list. Beware of the term "All Natural;" it does not mean organic. There are absolutely no regulations governing the use of this term by companies. It may contain the absolutely worst combination of GMO foods and other toxic ingredients and still be called "All Natural."

PFH Action Point

- **Eat organic produce when possible**
- **Get the Dirty Dozen and Clean Fifteen lists from Environmental Working Group**
- **Eat organic meats to avoid GMO ingredients, hormones and routine antibiotics**
- **Eat organic packaged foods when necessary, but remember that they still can have wheat**
- **"All Natural" does not mean organic and it can contain GMO and toxic ingredients**

As part of our **anti-inflammatory lifestyle**, I have previously discussed the need to consume large amounts of antioxidants. This is necessary to neutralize Free Radicals that are attacking our cells and our DNA. If you recall, Free Radicals are generated from multiple sources including the environment and the toxins we are exposed to. Some Free Radicals are produced within our bodies in response to stress, exercise, and metabolism. Antioxidants block the process of oxidation by scavenging these Free Radicals, neutralizing them, and allowing them to be excreted from the body. Antioxidants become oxidized in the process and must be constantly replenished. Antioxidants include antioxidant nutrients, antioxidant enzymes, and others. The most abundant intracellular antioxidant is Glutathione, which is produced in several pathways, including the Methylation Pathway, which we will look at in more depth later.

Let us look at some of the antioxidant nutrients that are so important for you to consume. Vitamin E, known as Tocopherol, is a fat soluble vitamin. Vitamin E has numerous important effects in our body. It protects cell membranes and prevents oxidation of LDL cholesterol. Therefore, it is very important in the prevention of atherosclerotic cardiovascular disease. There are several forms of Tocopherol with Alpha Tocopherol being the most common that you will see in a vitamin supplement. Gamma Tocopherol is much more potent and a little more expensive.

Vitamin C, also known as Ascorbic Acid, is a water soluble vitamin. Vitamin C scavenges Free Radicals in cells and helps to regenerate Vitamin E. It is a very essential vitamin and deficiency results in a condition called Scurvy. Vitamin C only stays in the body a short period of time. If you are taking a Vitamin C supplement, it must be taken multiple times per day, as it will be quickly excreted. Combining Vitamin C with bioflavonoids will increase its longevity in the body.

Beta-carotene is a water-soluble antioxidant nutrient found in fruits and vegetables with an orange color, such as carrots and sweet potatoes. Beta-carotene neutralizes singlet oxygen and scavenges other Free Radicals in a low oxygen environment. Other antioxidant nutrients include Selenium, Manganese, and Zinc. These are trace minerals and form the active sites of several antioxidant enzymes (Glutathione Peroxidase).

Another important antioxidant is CoenzymeQ10, which goes by the names Ubiquinone and Ubiquinol. CoenzymeQ10 is essential for mitochondrial production of ATP, which is the energy our cells run on. CoenzymeQ10 is actually part of the final steps of ATP production.

It also protects cellular organelles from Free Radicals. CoenzymeQ10 levels drop as we get older and will become deficient due to improper nutrition as well as several medications, including statin drugs.

PQQ, which stands for Pyrroloquinoline Quinone, is also essential for the mitochondrial production of ATP and protects the mitochondria from Free Radical damage. Uric Acid, which is a product of DNA metabolism and is elevated in the condition called Gout, is also an antioxidant.

Most of the antioxidants that are consumed in our diet are contained in fruits and vegetables and are called Phytochemicals. The most potent of these are Flavonoids. They are also known as Bioflavonoids or Vitamin P. Besides having potent antioxidant activity, Flavonoids also have anti-allergic, anti-inflammatory, anti-microbial, and anti-cancer activity. The most potent Flavonoids are Epicatechin and Catechin. Others include Resveratrol, Quercitin, and Anthocyanins. It is important to eat a rainbow of colors in order to obtain a variety of antioxidants, as each has different functions and benefits. This includes red, orange, yellow, purple, blue, and green.

We can measure the antioxidant activity of a food or other substance using a standardized scientific method known as ORAC. This stands for Oxygen Radical Absorbance Capacity. Brunswick Labs developed ORAC and it is the gold standard used by the USDA and research institutions around the world. The latest version of this is ORAC 5.0 and it is a comprehensive assessment of the antioxidant capacity of foods and other substances against the 5 primary Free Radicals that affect human health. When examining ORAC scores, it is clear that we need a broad spectrum of activity from many different foods as each one may only neutralize one or two of these Free Radicals.

When examining the ORAC scores of various fruits and vegetables, unprocessed cocoa (which is not listed in the tables below) is the highest antioxidant vegetable or fruit in the world. There are also several other super fruits that are extremely high in their antioxidant capacity. When you combine some of these together, you obtain the highest antioxidant food in the world, effective against all five major Free Radicals that affect human health. Our super food drinks can meet this criteria if constructed thoughtfully.

The charts reproduced below show examples of fruits, vegetables, spices, nuts and beans and their ORAC values. Not everything is included, especially some of the more exotic foods.

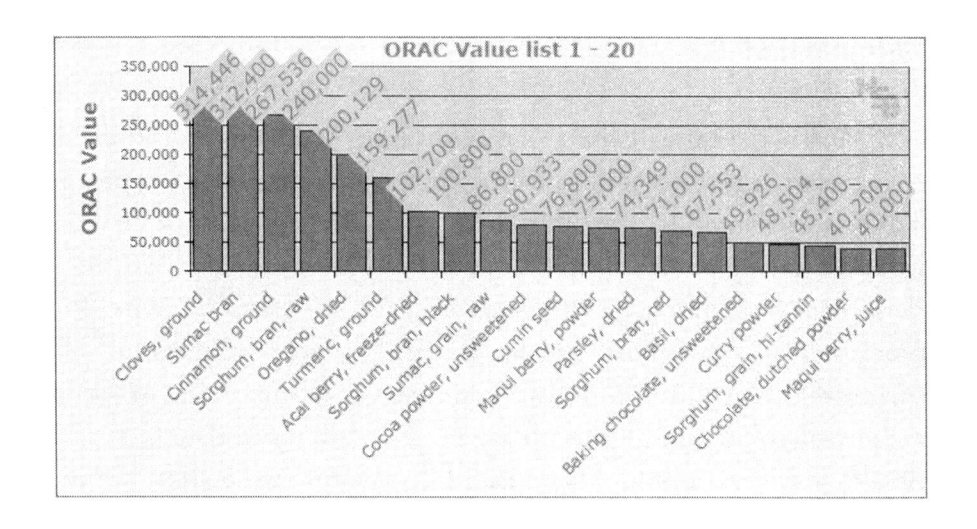

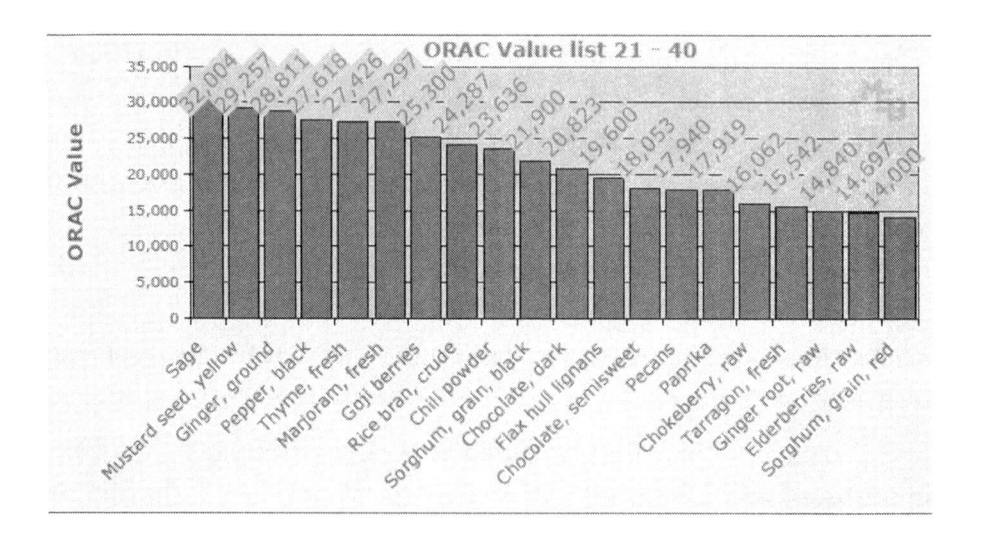

ORAC Value list 1 - 20

Food	ORAC Value
Cloves, ground	314,446
Sumac bran	312,400
Cinnamon, ground	267,536
Sorghum, bran, raw	240,000
Oregano, dried	200,129
Turmeric, ground	159,277
Acai berry, freeze-dried	102,700
Sorghum, bran, black	100,800
Sumac, grain, raw	86,800
Cocoa powder, unsweetened	80,933
Cumin seed	76,800
Maqui berry, powder	75,000
Parsley, dried	74,349
Sorghum, bran, red	71,000
Basil, dried	67,553
Baking chocolate, unsweetened	49,926
Curry powder	48,504
Sorghum, grain, hi-tannin	45,400
Chocolate, dutched powder	40,200
Maqui berry, juice	40,000

ORAC Value list 21 - 40

Food	ORAC Value
Sage	32,004
Mustard seed, yellow	29,257
Ginger, ground	28,811
Pepper, black	27,618
Thyme, fresh	27,426
Marjoram, fresh	27,297
Goji berries	25,300
Rice bran, crude	24,287
Chili powder	23,636
Sorghum, grain, black	21,900
Chocolate, dark	20,823
Flax hull lignans	19,600
Chocolate, semisweet	18,053
Pecans	17,940
Paprika	17,919
Chokeberry, raw	16,062
Tarragon, fresh	15,542
Ginger root, raw	14,840
Elderberries, raw	14,697
Sorghum, grain, red	14,000

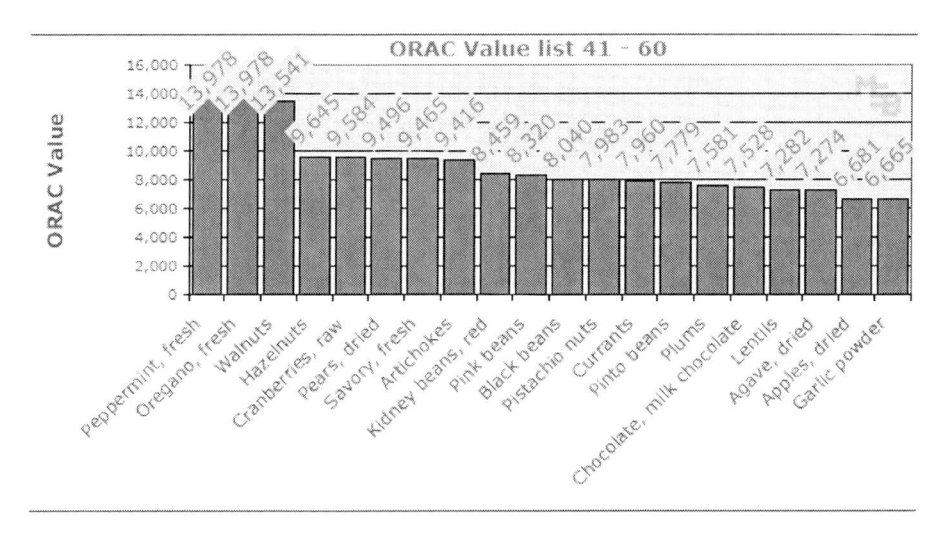

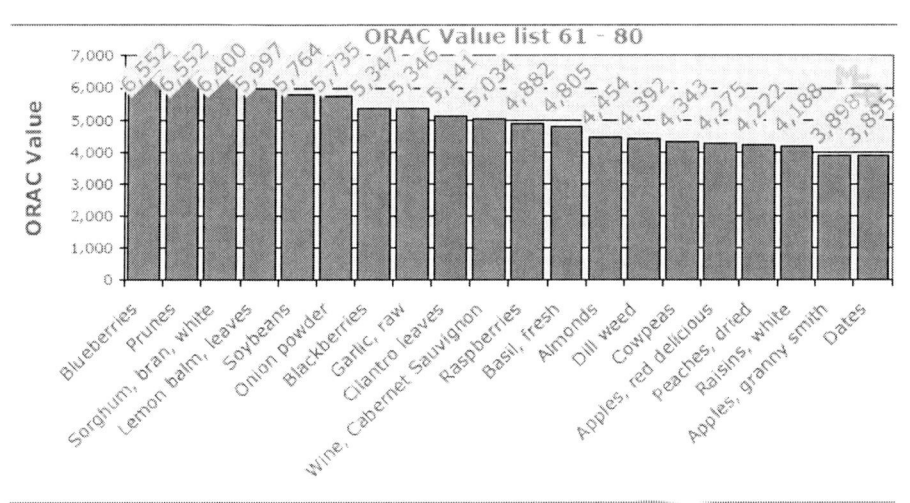

The highest antioxidant-rich foods are spices. The best include cloves, cinnamon, oregano, turmeric, cumin, parsley, basil, and curry. Try to include these when preparing your food or smoothie.

The highest antioxidant-rich fruits are Acai berries, Maqui berries, Goji berries, Chokeberries, Elderberries, Cranberries, Plums, Blueberries and Prunes. Consume them raw, dried, in your smoothies, or in recipes. Since it is hard to obtain many of these in their raw, organic form at the store, it is best to get them freeze dried or cold processed on the internet as powders to add to your recipes. Prunes are not just good for constipation after all.

The highest antioxidant-rich vegetables include unprocessed cocoa and Moringa. Neither are on these charts, but cocoa is in the top 5 and Moringa in the top 20. Moringa is a plant grown in other countries, including India and third world countries. It is highly nutritious. Other desirable vegetables include artichokes, garlic, red cabbage, kale, spinach, broccoli, red leaf lettuce, and beets.

Other high antioxidant-rich foods include nuts and seeds. The best are pecans, walnuts, hazelnuts, pistachios, almonds and sunflower seeds. The best beans are kidney, black, pinto, and soy. Lentils are also good. The best beverages are espresso, coffee, green tea, red wine, and fruit juices like acai and pomegranate. The down side of the juices is the sugar and calorie content.

As you proceed through these ORAC tables, you notice that common fruits and vegetables that we eat daily have much lower ORAC scores. Becoming familiar with this ORAC chart can be very helpful, as it will assist you in making decisions about what types of food to eat that will have the greatest health benefits. Remember that the antioxidant capacity will be improved if you consume these substances in their organic form, grown in organic soil and free of toxic pesticides.

PFH Action Point

- **We need to purposely consume antioxidants in our diet to fight Free Radicals**
- **Vitamin E, C, Beta Carotene, CoQ 10 and PQQ are important antioxidants**
- **Phytochemicals in fruits and vegetables, such as Flavonoids, are important to consume**
- **Focus on eating a rainbow of colors to obtain a variety of antioxidants**
- **Using the ORAC score and chart can help you make decisions about what to eat**

Let us focus on unprocessed cocoa since it is the highest antioxidant fruit or vegetable in the world. Cocoa has the highest concentration of Flavonoids of any food on the earth. It also has the highest ORAC score and ORAC 5.0 scores of any fruit or vegetable on the earth, meaning that it has a broad spectrum of activity against the 5 primary Free Radicals. This is not true of nearly every other antioxidant food. This broad spectrum of activity against Free Radicals is extremely helpful in our quest for an **anti-inflammatory lifestyle**. We are referring to unprocessed cocoa. We will go into detail about that shortly.

Unprocessed cocoa has many additional health benefits. It is high in good fatty acids such as Omega 3's. It contains much soluble and insoluble fiber, which is extremely important for your colon health. Cocoa contains a lot of magnesium, potassium, copper, iron, zinc and calcium. Given the nutrient deficiencies we commonly encounter in our nation, cocoa can be a great source of nutrient replacement. Any way that you look at it, cocoa is a medical super food and it tastes good!

The antioxidants in cocoa include Epicatchin and Catechin, which we looked at previously, and are some of the most powerful antioxidants known. Cocoa also contains Quercetin in similar concentrations as broccoli, apples, and red grapes. Cocoa also contains Resveratrol in concentrations roughly half as much as California Red Wine. It should be noted that up to 86% of these nutrients are lost in a process called Dutching. Many of the other nutrients, such as zinc, are also lost.

To understand the processing of cocoa, we must take a look at its history. Cocoa is from Cacao beans, originally discovered by the Aztec Indians in Mexico. Records show that they were consuming a drink made out of Cacao up to 3500 years ago. It was revered for its healing properties and healthful effects. When the Spanish came and conquered the Aztecs, they took Cacao beans back to Europe. However, the Cacao was fairly bitter and did not meet the taste expectations of the Europeans. In the nineteenth century, a process emerged called Dutching. The Cacao beans were melted in order to shape it into squares, circles, and other figurines for consumption. It was alkalized and heated to over 110 degrees, which destroys most of the antioxidants and enzymes in the cocoa. The cocoa

Butter was removed from the solids and was replaced with bad fats, refined sugars, caffeine, waxes, milk, coloring and fillers. The resulting chocolate made it less expensive to produce and tasted better to the populous, but robbed the cocoa of much of its beneficial health benefits.

In summary, one billion people will eat chocolate today. Americans consume 3 billion pounds of chocolate annually. In general, the chocolate we are eating is totally devoid of nutrients and is full of harmful fats, sugars, and fillers. This unhealthy chocolate is one of the major causes of our health crisis. Unprocessed cocoa is one of the healthiest foods on the earth. We must seek to eat unprocessed cocoa that contains the highest Cacao content and retains the original antioxidants. The cocoa I recommended in our discussion of super food smoothies meets those criteria. The chocolate that you are buying in the store does not.

PFH Action Point

- **Cocoa is the highest antioxidant fruit or vegetable on the earth**
- **It has a broad spectrum of antioxidant activity, making it very desirable to consume**
- **You must seek to eat cold processed cocoa as the nutrients are preserved; it is hard to find in stores and most store chocolate is dead and full of fats, sugars and fillers**
- **Cocoa also has omega 3's, fiber, and minerals**

Americans, in general, are very iron deficient. I see this all the time in my practice. I test all of my patients for iron levels. While I agree that I am seeing a select group of very sick patients, uniformly they are all iron deficient. And I am not just talking about a little. So why is iron deficiency running so rampant in America? I believe it has to do with a number of factors. Leaky Gut Syndrome is very common with the resultant poor absorption of nutrients. Toxins interfere with our ability to absorb nutrients. The food is being produced in nutrient depleted soil. Processed foods have had many of the nutrients removed.

Iron deficiency results in many health complications. While we all know that it creates anemia, this only happens when the deficiency gets really low. Iron is involved in many metabolic processes in our body. One of the important areas to me is how it affects thyroid function. Low iron levels definitely contribute to Hypothyroidism. It also has effects on our immune system, brain function, and energy production.

Below I have listed some top iron containing foods. It would be worthwhile to start making a conscious effort to consume more of these foods.

- Clams, oysters, mussels
- Dried pumpkin seeds; sesame and sunflower seeds
- Liver
- Dried apricots
- Sundried tomatoes
- Black Strap Molasses
- Spinach, Kale, and other dark greens
- Beef, shrimp, and dark meat turkey
- Beans and lentils
- Dried Thyme and Parsley
- Raw cocoa powder
- Cashews, Pine Nuts, and Almonds

PFH Action Point

- **Iron deficiency is common in America**
- **Causes are Leaky Gut, toxins, and nutrient depleted foods**
- **It results in anemia and contributes to Hypothyroidism, immune dysfunction, brain fog and fatigue**
- **Know the high iron-containing foods and focus on eating more of them**

As part of our **anti-inflammatory lifestyle**, it is extremely important to eliminate processed foods. Generally, processed foods are full of wheat, HFCS, and sugars. They often contain GMO ingredients. Scanning through an ingredient list of a typical processed food, you will see things such as colors/dyes, artificial flavors, preservatives, chemicals that you can't pronounce, fillers, and other toxins. I believe it is best to believe that if you cannot pronounce an ingredient, it is probably not good for you. In processed foods, many of the essential nutrients have been removed in the processing. They are generally full of empty calories.

Many of us resort to processed foods when we are looking for something to snack on. One of the worst is microwave popcorn. We have looked at this previously as it contains a large number of toxic substances. There are very high rates of cancers in those who work in plants producing microwave popcorn. When looking for a snack, try popping your own organic popcorn in a stainless steel skillet utilizing organic oil. You can also use organic blue corn tortilla chips that have less than three ingredients. Organic raw nuts are great. Another good snack is a small piece of organic fruit. You can also make one of our super food smoothies or other snack/dessert recipes containing these super foods.

Recently, Environmental Working Group came out with their long awaited Food Scores. They have an app for your smart phone that you can use to scan a food's barcode and get a summary of what things are in it. There is a score comparing it to other foods on a scale from 1 to 10. They tell you about its nutrient levels and toxin concerns. It is a great guide and a help to us as we seek to eliminate harmful and questionable foods from our diet.

It is essential that we avoid fast food in general. For the most part, fast foods are highly processed and devoid of many essential nutrients. They are high in saturated fats and bad carbohydrates. It seems that wheat is the essential focus of the meal. HFCS is in the food and the drinks. Fast foods generally contain too much salt, MSG, and other "natural flavorings." They are generally fried in rancid oils high in bad fatty acids. Fast foods are loaded with calories. In fact, one meal can easily be over 2,000 calories! They have been designed to suppress the production of grehlin, so that you can't tell that you are filled and want to keep eating.

PFH Action Point

- **Processed and fast foods need to be eliminated**
- **They are full of wheat, HFCS, and sugars**
- **They contain GMO ingredients, toxins, chemicals, preservatives, and artificial colors and flavors**
- **Use healthy snacks like fruit, nuts, organic popcorn, organic tortilla chips, and smoothies**
- **Use EWG's Food Scores to make decisions about what is safe to eat**

It is essential that we eliminate all rice from our diets. Consumer Reports did extensive testing of rice and rice products in November of 2012. They found that all United States rice was contaminated with Arsenic, most at levels far above what municipal water supplies are allowed. How did this contamination with Arsenic happen? The original land that rice is currently grown on was oftentimes used to raise tobacco crops. The pesticide that was sprayed on tobacco crops was very high in Arsenic. This Arsenic got into the soil and is still there today. Since rice highly concentrates water from the soil, the Arsenic is also being concentrated into the rice.

The report found that rice from other countries was far better. White rice from California had less Arsenic than other areas of the US. While we normally think that brown rice is healthier for us than white rice, it actually contains more Arsenic than white rice. Organic rice was found to be just as bad as nonorganic rice. The Arsenic problem also includes all products that are made from rice including rice syrup, rice solids, and rice milk. Remember that Arsenic has also been found in high concentrations in apple and grape juice and they should be avoided as well, especially in children.

It is important to remember, as part of our **anti-inflammatory lifestyle**, to avoid eating canned tuna and other sources of mercury. Consumer Reports did an excellent report of canned tuna in January 2011. They found that mercury levels were dangerously high in most tuna. In fact, albacore, which we usually consider to be a higher quality tuna, had higher levels of mercury than "chunk light." All of the tuna contained higher levels of mercury than would be safe to consume by anyone, especially pregnant women.

Canned salmon was found to have very low levels of mercury. However, remember to consider the BPA that is lining all of the cans and is another potent Endocrine Disruptor. Other fish that are high in mercury should be avoided including tuna steaks, swordfish, shark, mackerel, grouper, Chilean seabass, and orange roughy. You may be able to have one of these fish on a very rare basis, but never if you are pregnant.

PFH Action Point

- **Limit consumption of rice and rice products due to Arsenic contamination**
- **White rice from California or other countries has less Arsenic**
- **Avoid apple and grape juice due to Arsenic contamination**
- **Avoid all canned tuna as it is high in mercury and the cans have BPA**
- **Learn the other fish that are high in mercury and should be avoided**

There are a number of issues concerning the water that we consume. None of the nutrients and healthy foods that we have been discussing will work properly in our bodies if we are not consuming enough water. Most of the patients that I see are grossly dehydrated. In general, you need to be drinking half of your body weight in ounces per day of water. Most people are drinking far less than that. It is best to measure your intake of water utilizing a glass or stainless steel bottle where you already know the number of ounces that it contains. For example, I use a glass water bottle that contains 22 ounces. I know that if I have four of those per day, I am getting 88 ounces of water, which is more than half of my body weight. Dehydrated cells do not function properly and dehydrated tissues do not heal properly.

So what kind of water should we be drinking? We have looked extensively at the toxins that are found in our drinking water. It is clear that we must have a way to clean our water effectively to remove these toxins. The two methods that seem to do the best job are reverse osmosis and distilled. Tap water contains unacceptable levels of chlorine, fluoride, heavy metals, plastics, pesticides, pharmaceutical residues, and other potent Endocrine Disruptors. Reverse osmosis and distillation will remove virtually all of those things. Spring water still contains many contaminates and comes in plastic bottles.

An effective solution for generating clean water is to install a reverse osmosis unit under your kitchen sink. Some companies will even lease it to you for a small monthly charge. It will have a small faucet coming out next to your regular faucet. It generates enough water for a family to drink, cook with, and make ice with each day. While I agree with the purists who say it is best to install a unit on your entire house, finances are a consideration for most of us. Remember not to drink out of plastic water bottles as these contain high levels of plastics dissolved in the water. As for alkaline water, I have nothing against it, but do not believe that most people need it. It is best to repair body acidity through our **anti-inflammatory lifestyle**.

As for coffee and tea, recent studies have confirmed that there are significant antioxidants in both coffee and tea, including herbal teas. It is best to buy them in their organic form in order to eliminate pesticide contamination. They should be consumed in small to moderate amounts. Beware of the effects of the caffeine as a little is ok, but a lot is detrimental. There are lots of studies coming out showing that low dose consumption of coffee and tea can improve your lifespan and your cognitive functions. What you put in your coffee and tea is another matter. You must avoid artificial sweeteners, creamers, and sugars. It is best to use Stevia, Agave Nectar, honey, or some unprocessed pure cane sugar. Remember that coffee and tea consumption are not a replacement for your daily requirement of water. In fact, these substances can be dehydrating requiring even more water consumption.

PFH Action Point

- **Most people are dehydrated; we need to consume half our body weight in ounces per day**
- **Use reverse osmosis or distilled water to remove toxins**
- **Avoid all plastic bottles and cups; use glass or stainless steel**
- **Coffee and tea contain antioxidants and modest consumption can be very healthy**[1]

Chapter 9
I Can't Sleep

Americans are tired. As I speak with patients every day and start to inquire about their sleep patterns, I am universally shocked and appalled at how little sleep people are getting on a daily basis. The human body was not designed to live on four or five hours of sleep. Insomnia and other sleep dysfunctions are a very common complaint in primary care practices. However, as you start asking questions to patients presenting for other problems, you find that many of them are not sleeping well. While some of it may have to do with the mattress, as the mattress manufacturers would lead you to believe on TV, I believe the issues are far deeper than that.

Why aren't we sleeping? There are several substances that can ruin our sleep pattern. Caffeine, commonly found in coffee, teas, energy drinks, sodas, and chocolate, is a very common culprit. It is amazing to me how anyone can sleep when they are drinking two pots of coffee a day and consuming twelve diet sodas daily. It is well known that consuming caffeine after mid-afternoon will affect your nighttime sleep quality. I believe that chronic caffeine use has profound effects on your sleep. In addition, the sugars, HFCS, artificial sweeteners, bromine, and other stimulants in these drinks also affect your brain and result in hyperactivity. Other substances that affect your sleep include alcohol, prescription medications, and over-the-counter medications. Just read the list of side effects for many of the medications you are taking and insomnia will be prominently displayed.

Americans are generally "wired." This means that their brain is constantly in a state of excitation. This includes stresses from finances, work, overloaded schedules, and complex relationships. It also includes stimulation overload from surfing the web, video games, social media, and violent movies. All of this makes it very difficult to wind down at the end of the day and turn your brain off. I know many people that stay up into all hours of the night on the internet, communicating on social media, and playing video games. Then they wonder why they can't sleep.

Americans are generally overworked due to our economic situation. Families are forced to work multiple jobs in order to pay their bills. The 40-hour work week is no longer normal. This is especially true for single mothers. How can you possibly get enough sleep when you are working two jobs, taking care of the kids, cooking, cleaning, going to soccer games, and trying to deal with various relationships? There are not enough hours in the day to then get 7 or 8 hours of sleep. This can also be true of the corporate executive who is commuting long distances and the salaried manager who is being asked to do more with less.

A related issue is social pressure. There is a general view out there in society, and in the media, that sleep is not necessary. It is portrayed as a tremendous waste of your time and is keeping you from doing other things. It is almost to the point that you feel guilty when you are sleeping 8 hours. You feel that you should be doing something else, like web browsing, social media, working more, doing sports, and hanging out with your friends. Sleep is not a waste of time. Sleep is an essential part of our health and healing.

Worry is a big cause of sleeplessness. It may be worry over health issues and sickness. It may be worry over paying the bills and financial stress. It may be fear of the unknown and coming life changes. It may be relational problems such as abuse, divorce, unfaithfulness, and unrealistic expectations. There may be worry about retirement, investments, the economy, and how you are going to survive. What about the work situation or the lack of work? You may be worried about all of the things that you have to do tomorrow and not having enough time to do them all. And there may be spiritual fears that have been left unresolved.

PFH Action Point
- **Insomnia is widespread in America**
- **Caffeine and other stimulants affect sleep, so use them sparingly**
- **Worry, stress, excessive work, and over-stimulation keep us "wired" and unable to sleep**
- **Society tells you that you don't need 7-8 hours of sleep, but you do**

There are a number of health issues that directly affect sleep. Obesity can be a significant cause of sleep dysfunction. Not only are there mechanical problems with pressure on the diaphragm, but it may be uncomfortable to even reposition yourself during the nighttime. Obesity can result in Obstructive Sleep Apnea (OSA) with resultant disruptive sleep from apnea episodes (stop breathing). Many find it very difficult to sleep while wearing the CPAP mask used to treat the OSA. Obesity and diabetes can cause blood sugar abnormalities during the nighttime, which will affect sleep.

Another medical condition affecting sleep is Restless Leg Syndrome (RLS). This is the feeling that your legs have to keep moving at nighttime and you have no control over them. This is very disruptive to sleep. If you have RLS, it is very important to avoid all caffeinated beverages and alcohol. Smoking must cease immediately. It is important to stretch and do relaxation exercises prior to bedtime. I have found that magnesium supplements are very helpful in reducing these symptoms. A related issue is leg cramps, which is treated in a similar fashion as RLS.

Nocturia is the term to describe frequent awakenings at nighttime to void. It is the number one cause of sleep disorders in older adults. Nocturia can be caused by prostate problems, such as Benign Prostatic Hypertrophy (BPH), irritable bladder, and elevated blood sugars. As we get older, less Anti-diuretic Hormone (ADH) is produced resulting in an inability to hold fluids in your body. This seems to be worse during the nighttime. If you have nocturia, it is important to limit fluids late at night. You must avoid all alcohol and caffeinated beverages. Citrus fruits have been shown to worsen this condition. Artificial sweeteners must be avoided entirely.

GERD (Gastro Esophageal Reflux Disease) can definitely affect the quality of sleep. GERD is a condition where acid will come up into the esophagus, from the stomach, due to a loosening of the sphincter at the bottom of the esophagus. There are a number of things that do affect GERD. It is definitely worse when lying down. It is important to stay upright three hours after you eat. Obesity contributes greatly to this disorder, so losing weight is paramount. Things that can affect this lower esophageal sphincter include alcohol, cigarettes, milk and dairy products, aspirin and anti-inflammatory medications, chocolate and some spicy/acidic/fatty foods. Some people complain that citrus fruits and tomatoes greatly affect their GERD. Antacids can be helpful temporarily. There are some natural treatments for GERD including products made from orange peel. MSM also seems to help. The medications commonly prescribed for GERD, especially the proton pump inhibitors, have numerous and significant side effects.

Another significant cause of sleeplessness is hot flashes. I deal a lot with women who complain that at nighttime they have all the sheets thrown off, the fan turned on, and they are sweating in their pillows while their husband is sound asleep under the covers. Hot flashes can be very debilitating. While they typically occur around the time of menopause, they can occur anytime a woman's hormones are significantly out of balance. Since Endocrine Disruptors cause these hormone imbalances, hot flashes can be a sign of significant toxicity. While the ultimate cure is to correct the underlying condition, there are several symptomatic treatments that seem to help. Evening Primrose Oil and Black Cohash are two natural supplements that seem to have some benefit in controlling symptoms. Ultimately, I have to test for hormone levels and balance those hormones in order to control these debilitating symptoms and improve the quality of sleep.

PFH Action Point

- **Obesity and Obstructive Sleep Apnea disrupt sleep patterns**
- **Restless Leg Syndrome and Nocturia keep people from sleeping**
- **GERD and hot flashes keep many up at night**
- **Treating the underlying problem is essential to getting a good night's sleep**

So how much sleep do we need? This is not an easy question to answer. However, it is clearly more than we are getting currently. If we look at our recent history, the average person in the United States in the year 1900 was getting 9 hours of sleep. One hundred plus years later, the average American now gets 6.5 hours of sleep. There is a sleep deficit of 2.5 hours over the last 100 years. What happened? And what have been the effects of this lack of sleep?

There are a lot of reasons why we are sleeping less than we did 100 years ago. We have identified some of those factors above. Add to that all of the distractions that we have competing for our attention in our daily lives. This includes TV, internet, cell phones, social media, video games, and other distractions. The result has been increasing poor health in our nation. Now while this poor health can be related to many factors that we have discussed already, sleep deprivation certainly contributes to it.

The average person needs somewhere between 7 to 9 hours of sleep. This depends very much on the individual. I know some people that seem to function quite optimally on 6 hours sleep. I know others that feel terrible unless they get 9 hours of sleep. I seem to function best at somewhere around 8 hours of sleep. The best guide seems to be that you sleep until you wake up without an alarm and feel refreshed. How many of us are actually doing that?

The quality of our sleep is also important. Now that we have had a lot of experience doing sleep studies, we understand more about sleep architecture. During the night, we move through sleep cycles numerous times. This includes REM sleep and non-REM sleep, which is divided into stages 1 through 4. Both REM and non-REM sleep are equally important in maintaining our physical and mental health. REM sleep is "active" sleep where dreams take place and our body systems resemble when we are awake. It is important for mental health. Non-REM sleep is where our body systems calm down and is important for physical health. Stages 1 and 2 are termed "light" sleep and stages 3 and 4 are termed "deep" sleep. Most healthy adults spend about 75% of their sleep time in non-REM and 25% in REM sleep. The first half of the night is usually non-REM sleep with brief periods of REM as we progress through sleep cycles about every 90 minutes. REM sleep reaches maximum in the last third of the night and non-REM stages 3 and 4 decrease.

It is important to spend a lot of time in stage 3 and 4 sleep because this is where our brain and body heal; the immune system is regenerated, brain chemicals are restored, hormone systems are rebalanced, muscles and other tissues begin to heal, and our ATP reservoirs are replenished. If you spend most of your night in light stages of sleep, such as REM or non-REM stages 1 and 2, much of this healing does not occur and you wake up feeling exhausted and fatigued. You wind up going through the day feeling tired with poor cognitive function and generally poor energy levels (Excessive Daytime Sedation or EDS). In order to compensate for that, most people resort to substances like caffeine, sugar, or chocolate to keep going.

This is a common finding in pain patients. People in pain will awaken a lot during the night and cycle back to non-REM stage 1 sleep without spending much time in stages 3 or 4. This only serves to perpetuate the pain by preventing restorative healing, both physically and mentally. The sleep deficit results in fatigue and an inability to cope with pain. The pain threshold is lowered and they experience more pain. This results in depression and more pain. They then seek to increase the use of pain medications, with resultant side effects and further effects on sleep. Opioid pain medications disrupt REM sleep and create an imbalance in sleep architecture, affecting mental health and resulting in more pain. It is a vicious cycle that can only be interrupted by addressing the sleep problem and the cause of the pain.

PFH Action Point

- **The average person needs 7-9 hours of sleep, depending on the individual**
- **Optimum is to sleep until wake up without an alarm**
- **Quality of sleep is very important; you need to move through several complete sleep cycles of REM and non-REM sleep each night**
- **Healing takes place during deep sleep, especially non-REM stages 3 and 4**

Sleep deprivation results in Excessive Daytime Sedation (EDS). EDS results in poor performance in work and school. It is also been correlated with motor vehicle accidents and worker's compensation injuries. Cognitive and motor functions become significantly impaired. EDS has been related to such disasters as the Challenger explosion, the Exxon Valdese oil spill, the 3 Mile Island nuclear plant disaster, and other notable mishaps. A good screening test for EDS is the Epworth Sleepiness Scale. A score above 10 indicates a significant sleep quality problem; the maximum is 24. It can be found online.

Sleep dysfunction is responsible for significant healthcare expenses in the United States. This includes sleep centers doing myriads of sleep studies on sleep-deprived people. Many times this results in a prescription for a CPAP machine to use at home during the nighttime. Many people will start using these and quickly abandon them because they do not like using them at nighttime for various reasons. There are expenses for oxygen therapy, home healthcare, and medical supplies. There are large expenditures for medications to help with the sleep dysfunction running rampant in our society. I have to admit that I have to use these sleep promoting agents on quite a few patients until I can get them feeling better and their sleep normalizes. Add to all of this the healthcare expenditures for the complications resulting from sleep deprivation, and it is clear that this is a significant portion of our healthcare dollars.

Sleep deprivation also results in several chronic diseases that we deal with in this country. It is clear that lack of sleep contributes to the development of diabetes, hypertension, cardiovascular disease, and stroke. Add together the additional healthcare expenses for these disorders, and it is clear that sleep deprivation is a financial drain on our society.

PFH Action Point

- **Sleep deprivation results in Excessive Daytime Sedation (EDS); the Epworth Sleepiness Scale is a good screening tool**
- **EDS causes poor work and school performance**
- **EDS results in accidents and injuries, costing money and bringing emotional upheavals**
- **Sleep deprivation results in huge economic losses in healthcare expenditures and lost business productivity**

So what can we do to improve our sleep? I will be looking here at some natural things that can help with sleep. The first is sleep hygiene. It is very important to avoid eating late at night and drinking fluids for several hours before bedtime as these may induce GERD or Nocturia. However, a bedtime snack of a small amount of protein can be helpful to stabilize your blood sugar throughout the night. Hypoglycemia can cause you to wake up and have difficulty falling back to sleep again. Your bedroom should be kept cool, quiet, and very dark. The temperature should be very comfortable, preferably a little on the cooler side.

There should be no loud noises in your bedroom. The exception would be if you have tinnitus, or ringing in the ears; in this case, having background noise will be very helpful to drown the tinnitus out. Some patients seem to do much better when there is background noise such as a fan, a sound machine with sounds of the seashore playing, or other calming background sounds. It is very important to turn off all lights and this includes those annoying LED lights that are on our electronic equipment. If you can't get the room quiet, say because of a snoring partner, earplugs can be very useful. If you can't get all of the light out of your room, then a nighttime eye covering can be very helpful.

It is important to wind down and turn off any media that you are watching a minimum of 30 minutes before you go to bed. You should never watch television while sitting in bed. It is important to program your brain that the bed is for sleep. Therefore, when you go to bed, your brain will be expecting to go to sleep. If you watch TV in bed, your brain will be confused. Reading in bed does not seem to have that kind of affect and can be very calming prior to bedtime. I prefer to read the Bible before going to bed, especially something in the Psalms, as I find it very calming for my brain.

Exercise definitely improves the quality of your sleep. This includes both aerobic and non-aerobic exercise. It is important to do this exercise earlier in the day as exercise done just prior to bedtime will often interfere with your ability to go to sleep. For those having trouble turning their brain off at bedtime, I suggest keeping a pad/pen next to the bed and making a list of all of the things that you are worried about or thinking about so that you don't keep focusing on them. Oftentimes, I find myself lying in bed thinking about things that I need to do the next day and being afraid that I will forget to do them. By making a list, I no longer have to think about them. For those totally unable to turn their brain off at night, cognitive behavioral therapy can be useful.

The subject of naps during the daytime can be controversial. Numerous cultures take a nap in the early to mid-afternoon and have been doing that for thousands of years. This time period generally corresponds with a decline in our Cortisol levels and a post-prandial lack of energy as our body works on digesting our lunch. Studies show that a power nap of only 30 minutes or so can be very helpful. Naps longer than an hour will disturb your nighttime sleep architecture. I wish I had the time to take a nap every day about 2 o'clock. The times that I am able to lie down and sleep for even 15 minutes significantly rejuvenate me for the rest of the day.

PFH Action Point

- **Proper sleep hygiene is essential to regular, refreshing sleep**
- **Your room should be dark, cool and quiet; you may need earplugs or an eye covering**
- **Turn off your brain prior to bedtime; make a list of things you are worried about and try reading the Bible or another good book**
- **Exercise helps sleep, but should be done earlier in the day**
- **Naps can be useful, but only less than an hour or you will affect night time sleep**

There are several supplements that I utilize for people that are having trouble sleeping. For those that are having trouble falling asleep, I recommend a sustained release Melatonin, usually 5 milligrams, to take 2 hours prior to bedtime. Melatonin is a hormone produced in the brain that tells your brain that it is time to go to sleep. Since it is generally released several hours prior to your normal sleep time, it would be best to take it then. Many people are deficient in Melatonin production. This includes Biotoxin patients that we have discussed earlier.

If you are having trouble turning your brain off, taking Theanine 1 to 2 hours prior to bedtime can be helpful. Theanine is an extract from green tea and increases levels of GABA in the brain. GABA is one of the calming neurotransmitters. 200 milligrams of Theanine is a good dose. Since Theanine is calming to the brain and generally safe, you can use it every 8 hours when feeling stressed or anxious. In addition, Taurine 1000 milligrams is very calming. It regulates the relationship between the excitatory and calming neurotransmitters in the brain. Specifically, it helps to lower levels of Glutamate, which is an excitatory chemical in the brain. Again, taking Taurine 1 to 2 hours before bedtime is helpful.

Other supplements that are helpful for sleep include Tryptophan 500 milligrams, which is the same amino acid that is in turkey and makes us feel tired after a turkey dinner. Tryptophan is one of the precursors in the manufacture of Serotonin in our brain. Serotonin is also one of the calming neurotransmitters. 5-HTP is also a precursor of Serotonin and some people prefer to take that instead. Another supplement that can be useful is Phosphatidylserine (PS) 100 to 300 milligrams as this will help to bring down Cortisol levels and calm the brain. Rhodiola extract is an Adrenal Adaptogen and also helps to lower Cortisol levels and reduce stress. Many people use Valerian Root to help induce sleep. However, Valerian has some stimulation of opioid receptors and therefore acts like a weak narcotic. There have been reports of dependence with chronic use. Occasional use may be perfectly safe. I have shied away from using Valerian Root with my patients.

If natural supplements are not helping with your sleep, especially if you wake up in the middle of the night and can't get back to sleep, then medications may be necessary until the underlying condition is corrected. I will not go into the various medications that can be used for sleep in this book as their indications depend on the patient's problem, other medications, illnesses, age, and addiction potential.

If you snore, especially if you snore loudly, you may be at risk for apnea episodes. Apnea means to stop breathing. It is not unusual to stop breathing at times during the night for several seconds. However, if your spouse has to hit you to wake you up so you can breathe, there is a problem. It is important to ask your spouse if you are having episodes where you stop breathing for many seconds. Generally, people with apnea episodes will have frequent nighttime awakenings. If this is occurring, especially if you experience EDS, it is important to have a sleep study performed by a qualified sleep center. It is then important to follow up with a physician who is a certified sleep specialist.

PFH Action Point

- **Supplements that can help with sleep include Melatonin, which helps initiate sleep**
- **Theanine increases GABA and Taurine decreases Glutamate to calm the brain**

- **Tryptophan and 5-HTP help to make Serotonin to reduce anxiety**
- **Rhodiola and Phospatidlyserine help sleep by acting to lower Cortisol**
- **If you snore loudly, have apnea episodes, or have frequent nighttime awakenings and have EDS, you need a sleep study**

A related topic is the concept of stress reduction. Since it seems that our stressful lives affect our sleep and health in general, it seems appropriate now to talk about how to reduce stress in our lives. There will always be stress in our society, and it does not seem like it will be getting less over time. All indications are that we are living in a progressively more stressful world each year. There are a few concepts that I think are important to manage your stress.

The first concept is of creating margin in your life. We seem to all just be running from one thing to the next thing without any time to breathe. The concept of margin is creating space in your life to sit and rest and take some time for yourself and with God. I know that in my own case, I have to schedule this margin in my life. If I don't schedule it, it does not seem to happen. This includes my daily Quiet Time with God, exercise, sleep, and other quiet activities. Scheduling margin in your life is critically important for your physical and mental health. God knew this when He gave the 10 Commandments and told us to set aside one day weekly to rest, the Sabbath Day. It must be important to take time to rest, because God did it on the seventh day of creation.

Another concept of equal importance is the idea of boundaries. This involves knowing when to say "no." How is it that one of the first words a child says is "no" and they seem to have no problem saying it? Why can't adults say "no"? The "no" word can be very hard to say for those of us that are people pleasers, try to fix everyone, or have a natural desire to help others. Some people have a very hard time saying no. I used to be one of them.

When I ran the Emergency Department, everyone came to me with their problems because they knew that Dr. Gruning would take care of it. And I did, because I mistakenly believed that I could do the work better than everyone else, so it was less of a hassle to do it myself than to clean up someone else's mess. By enabling the staff, they never reached their full potential and I was left with no time to ever get caught up and have some margin in my life.

When I learned about setting boundaries, it was a very hard transition. I started slowly, by delegating tasks that were not essential to others. I then progressed to empowering others to fix their own problems with some guidance from me. Then I just started saying no, in a nice way, to requests that did not really need my involvement.

Eventually, I got to the hard part. I made a list of everything that I did in a given week, from the mundane to the important. Some of these were very good things, like involvement with my family, certain church and ministry activities, and civic organizations. I started drawing a line through everything that was not a top priority. My priorities were my relationship with Jesus, my family, my job and ministry. I then got on the phone and started calling people, letting them know that I would no longer be doing those things due to a lack of time. It was very freeing. Now, I do this every few months. Busyness has a way of creeping back in.

The best way I have found to reduce stress is to take to heart what the Apostle Paul told us in Philippians 4:6-7: *Be anxious for nothing, but in everything by prayer and supplication with thanksgiving let your requests be made known to God. And the peace of God, which surpasses all comprehension, will guard your hearts and your minds in Christ Jesus.*

I have successfully put this into practice in my life and I hope you will, too. I have used this passage of scripture with countless anxious and stressed out patients over the years. Those who listened and put into practice what it says have felt much better. Those who did not, continued to be anxious and often wound up on medications.

What Paul is saying is that we are not to be anxious, about anything! Now, if anyone had cause to be anxious, it was Paul. He was constantly under threat of persecution, death, financial problems, health issues, relationship problems, and churches that we were having troubles. What was his solution? He says that if we have a relationship with God through Jesus Christ we have no reason to be anxious. God is still on the throne and He is in control. He is the Most High (El Elyon), the Lord of Hosts (Yahweh Sabaoth), the Almighty God (El Shaddai) Who owns it all and controls it all. Nothing can come our way without His permission. It is all happening according to His will, so stressing about it accomplishes nothing.

Paul says the cure to anxiety and worry is to pray. Pray about everything. Bring your requests to God. Let them go. Don't dwell on your problems. Supplication means to really surrender the need to the Lord and earnestly seek His will to be done; this is not just a casual prayer. It is best to do this on your knees or on your face. Lay them at the foot of the cross and leave them there.

Paul goes on to say that you should give thanks. It is hard to be anxious about things when you are thanking God for everything you have instead of worrying about what you don't have. He is our Provider (Jehovah-jireh), our Protector (Jehovah-nissi), our Deliverer and He is our All Sufficient God. Our God is so Faithful (El Emmunah). He knows what we need and He will take care of it for us.

Paul goes on to say that for those that practice this, who pray and give thanks, the peace of God is theirs to rest in. This peace is beyond your understanding and logic and will guard your heart and mind in Christ Jesus. A peace will come over you that you can't understand or explain. That peace will guard your heart, which is the source of emotions, and your mind, which is the source of your thoughts. Only God can supply this peace. The world can't bring peace. It brings only stress. If you don't have this peace of God in your life, perhaps it is time for you to explore where you are in your spiritual life. We will talk more about that in our last chapter. There is also an Appendix with God's Promises. Read them and take them to heart. You won't be anxious any more.

I Can't Sleep

This time of prayer is part of a daily Quiet Time or Devotion Time with God. It has been a daily part of my life since 1991. It is a time to spend alone with your Heavenly Father. It is a time to pray, as we discussed, and to read God's Word, the Bible. It must be done in a quiet place and you need to schedule the time or it won't happen. I do my Quiet Time early in the morning, before the day begins. It can be in your room, a study, out in the woods, on the beach, wherever you can get alone with God and undisturbed. Turn off the TV, internet, phones, and all the distractions. You need to get quiet to hear God's voice.

Perhaps make a plan to read the Bible each year. It only takes 15 minutes per day. Do you know that only a small percent of Christians have ever read the whole Bible? There are great devotionals and phone apps to help with that, to keep you on track. I have read the Bible each year for many years now and can tell you that it brings everything together so that you can better see who God is, how He works, and what He wants you to know and do. The Holy Spirit teaches you as you read the scriptures and helps you to change your life. It is a powerful time.

PFH Action Point

- **Stress and anxiety permeate our society and rob us of peace**
- **Creating margin and setting boundaries are effective tools to manage stress**
- **Following Paul's words in Philippians 4:6-7 is an effective cure to anxiety and worry**
- **Having a daily Quiet Time with God will change your life for the better**

Chapter 10
ELIMINATING THE TOXINS

As I described in an earlier chapter, we are living in a chemical soup. Toxins are all around us, lurking in our air, food, water, personal care products, medications, and household products. In order to survive and flourish in this toxic world, we all must make a determined, conscious effort to eliminate as many of these toxins as we can. Let us take a look at how to do this.

First, understand that all of this attention to nutrition, lifestyle changes and toxin elimination is designed to adopt an **anti-inflammatory lifestyle**. None of this will be effective if we continue to poison our bodies with tobacco, alcohol and drugs. When I was working as an Emergency Physician, it was obvious to all of us that we spent half of our time cleaning up the mess caused by these substances. Whether directly or indirectly, half of our health care expenditures, hospitalizations, medications, treatments, and office visits are related to the abuse of these substances.

Everyone today knows that cigarette smoking causes cancer and Cardiovascular disease. We have been teaching it in the schools for decades and there are warnings on the packages. We don't need to review that. However, there are other effects of tobacco use that are not as obvious.

Tobacco use affects pituitary, thyroid, adrenal, testicular and ovarian function. Tobacco products directly alter the production and effect of the hormones produced by these essential organs. It also affects

Calcium metabolism, causing Osteoporosis. We are seeing an epidemic of Osteoporosis and it is occurring at younger ages. Tobacco use creates insulin resistance, a major reason for the development of diabetes. It also is a toxin that produces Free Radicals in our bodies, thus triggering Auto-immune diseases. Tobacco use results in low oxygen levels in the blood and tissues of our bodies (Hypoxemia) and replaces that oxygen with Carbon Monoxide, a cellular poison. Our tissues are literally starved for oxygen. These tissues are then prone to disease and can't repair when damaged.

Since no one will ever get better from their inflammatory lifestyle while continuing to use tobacco products, it is essential to quit using them immediately. I realize this is easier said than done. I have been dealing with addictions and addicted people my entire medical career. Every addict tells me it is easier to quit many of the drugs they use than to quit smoking. It is a terrible habit and it is readily available. However, if we are to adopt this new **anti-inflammatory lifestyle**, smoking and other forms of tobacco use have to go.

I have tried every possible way to get people off of cigarettes. I have prescribed gum, patches, pills, nasal sprays, and you name it. I have patients using e-cigs and they still continue smoking. It is apparent that if you want to quit, you will and the method does not seem to matter. If you don't want to quit, you won't despite the method used.

The most successful method for quitting smoking is actual a Scripture substitution program. A church developed this method, but anyone can use it. It does not cost a fortune and it is easily used by everyone. First, you must understand that in any addiction, you are powerless to fix it. The Twelve Steps used by Alcoholics Anonymous have verified this over the years. As originally developed by the founders of AA, this was a Christian organization that recognized that it was only by the power of Christ that any addiction could be overcome. You have to admit you have a problem, that you are powerless to overcome it, and that you need Jesus to do it for you (now it is a higher power). On your own, you cannot sustain a recovery from substances. This is a spiritual battle with the forces of darkness that want to enslave us and ruin our lives.

In tobacco addiction, the program works by getting index cards, say 20 or 30 of them, and writing meaningful Bible verses on them. An example would be Philippians 4:17: *I can do all things through Christ who gives me the strength.* You place the index cards where you would normally carry your cigarettes. Whenever you feel the urge to smoke, you take out your Bible verses and read them out loud and claim victory over the addiction. You can say something like, "Lord, I am powerless over this addiction. I need You to take away the desire to smoke, in Jesus' Name." By giving the problem to the Lord, you are doing what Jesus said. He wants you to cast your burdens upon Him. He is bigger than any problem you face. Obviously, this only works if you have a relationship with Jesus. Perhaps that is the next step for you. You can go to the Appendix to find helpful promises in God's Word and explore how to have a relationship with Jesus Christ.

One thing that I encounter all the time among Christians is a misunderstanding of how the Lord works in addictions. Most believe that they can pray a prayer and Jesus will arrive at their door and take the offending addiction away, in this case, all the cigarettes. That is not how it works. You have to surrender the addiction to Him and then ask for His help. That means making a commitment to quit and demonstrating that by getting rid of all the cigarettes. A good way to do that is to gather them up from wherever you have them hidden and put them in a bucket of water, pledging to not buy any more of them. Think of all the money you will save. I am shocked at how much money seemingly committed Christians spend on cigarettes, alcohol or other addictive drugs and then don't have enough money to give toward ministries that are doing the Lord's work. This should not be happening in your life.

Alcohol use and abuse is a scourge that destroys people and families. Again, I have been dealing with alcoholics my entire medical career. It is a terrible addiction to try to beat. I am not opposed to someone having an occasional glass of wine or beer. I have chosen not to drink alcohol. I think there are numerous Bible verses that admonish us not to use it for health reasons that have borne out to be true over time. More importantly, I do not want to cause a weaker brother to stumble into alcohol because of my tacit endorsement. You never know if they have a genetic predisposition to alcoholism because of their ability to metabolize alcohol differently than the rest of us. It is between you and the Lord if you want to have an occasional drink. However, when you need to have a drink, or others say that you have a problem with alcohol, then it has become a stronghold in your life and it needs to go.

I have had many patients tell me that they drink red wine at dinner daily because their doctor said it was good for them based on studies. Yes, red wine in small amounts is part of the Mediterranean Diet. However, where does the benefit come from? It is not the alcohol in the wine that provides the health benefits, that much is very clear. You can get the same health benefits from drinking red grape juice. It is from the Resveratrol in the grapes, a potent and well-studied antioxidant. You can get more Resveratrol from raw organic cocoa than wine. It is not worth the negative effects of the alcohol to consume wine daily.

Not only does alcohol use cause liver diseases like cirrhosis and liver cancer, but it has numerous other health consequences. Alcohol use can directly cause Hypothyroidism, Hormone Imbalances, menstrual problems and infertility. It has been linked to the development of breast cancer, osteoporosis and diabetes. Alcohol poisons the gut and causes Leaky Gut Syndrome, resulting in the malabsorption of nutrients like magnesium, iron, and potassium. As we have seen, alcohol is metabolized into fat by the Liver and causes atherosclerosis by increasing Triglycerides and oxidizing LDL cholesterol.

Drugs are another scourge on families and society. How many families have you known who were traumatized by a drug user, often a child. While the metabolic and inflammatory results of using drugs are beyond the scope of this book, suffice it to say that they are not good for an **anti-inflammatory lifestyle**.

With the advent of the legalization of marijuana, often disguised as something needed for medical reasons, people seem to have forgotten what a profoundly harmful drug pot is. While I don't need to prescribe it, we have had the opportunity to prescribe medical marijuana for cancer patients and others needing it for some time now. We don't need new laws for that. Marijuana is the gateway drug that every drug addict will tell you they started with. It damages the cells and chemicals of your brain and causes cognitive dysfunction, personality disturbances, and psychological pathology. It causes hormone imbalances and men can be seen growing breasts commonly (it does not do the same for women). Add to that the toll from impaired drivers and work related accidents, and it is hard to justify its use for the vast majority of us seeking to live a healthier life.

PFH Action Point

- **Toxin elimination is an essential part of our anti-inflammatory lifestyle**
- **All tobacco products must be eliminated**
- **Alcohol is a poison and should not be consumed except is small amounts occasionally**
- **Red wine is part of the Mediterranean Diet, but the health benefits come from the Resveratrol in the grape juice**
- **Drugs, including marijuana, are not part of our new lifestyle and must go**

Another class of toxins that we need to look at is called Goitrogens. These are toxins that interfere with thyroid function by either preventing iodine uptake (thyroid hormone is made from iodine) or by interfering with the conversion of T4 (inactive thyroid hormone) to T3 (active thyroid hormone). Thyroid hormone controls your metabolism and has many interactions with other body hormones and pathways. When not enough is made, or there is a lack of the active Free T3, Hypothyroidism results. We will look at thyroid diseases and thyroid support in more detail later.

A group of chemicals we need to look at are called Halogens. This goes back to basic chemistry class. The Halogens are chlorine, fluoride, bromine and iodine. They all have a negative charge. Unfortunately, the

Halogens can all compete for the same thyroid receptors and the non-iodine Halogens will block the use of iodine by the thyroid to make T4. The non-iodine Halogens can also interfere with T4 to T3 conversion.

Chlorine is a Goitrogen that is found in your drinking water, of all places. In fact, in many public water supplies, the amount of chlorine in the drinking water is the same as that in a typical pool. Just use a pool testing kit for yourself and see. You are drinking this chlorine into your body and it is interfering with your thyroid function. Chlorine is also present in high concentrations in public pools and is absorbed through your skin. It is essential to have a high quality water purification system to remove this toxin from your water. Reverse osmosis water or distilled are the best as they remove most other toxins as well. Pools can be maintained without chlorine by utilizing ozone-generating systems or by using salt water.

Fluoride is a Goitrogen that is found in your drinking water in the United States. It was put there after studies by dentists showed that it reduced tooth decay. Most other industrialized nations have chosen to either not fluoridate their water or to stop doing it. Why does the United States still insist on putting this thyroid toxin in our water? There are other ways to prevent tooth decay, like restricting sugar intake in beverages and foods and consuming more antioxidants. You need to remove it from your drinking water by using reverse osmosis or distilled water. Fluoride is also found in most toothpaste and we tend to swallow a lot of it, especially children. It is easier to find Fluoride-free toothpastes now, even in your local grocery store or pharmacy. Get rid of the Fluoride toothpastes.

Bromine is a Goitrogen that is present in wheat flour in the US. How did this happen? Prior to the 1980's, iodine was used as a de-caking agent in wheat flour. The chemical industry successfully lobbied the FDA to replace it with Bromine due to an iodine phobia that had developed due to a few faulty studies. Follow the money. It is very hard to find wheat flour without Bromine, so this is another reason to eliminate wheat from your diet. Bromine is also found commonly in hot tubs. Some people use chlorine. With the high heat, the Bromine and chlorine are aerosolized and you breathe it in, absorbing it through your lungs as well as your skin. Alternative methods to keep the hot tub clean include using ozone generators with non-chlorine shock and using salt water.

Other Goitrogens include plastics like PCB's and pesticides like DDT. These directly interfere with thyroid function. Nitrates in fertilizers are also toxic to your thyroid. Lithium, often used as an inexpensive pharmaceutical treatment for Bipolar Disorder, is toxic to the thyroid. Polycyclic hydrocarbons are also Goitrogens.

PFH Action Point
- **Goitrogens are toxic to the thyroid gland**
- **Chlorine is in drinking water and pools and must be eliminated**
- **Fluoride is in drinking water and toothpaste and must be avoided**
- **Bromine is in wheat flour and hot tubs and must be avoided**
- **Other Goitrogens include plastics, pesticides, nitrates, Lithium, and polycyclic hydrocarbons**

We have looked at many toxins in previous chapters, but let me review some of the high points with you. The world of Persistent Organic Pollutants (POP's) is extensive and includes plastics, pesticides and other Endocrine Disruptors. These are so named because they disrupt the way your Endocrine, Immune and Neurologic systems work.

Plastics include PCB's, Dioxin, BPA, and Phthalates. They are found in many common products, including foods and supplements. You must be diligent to eliminate plastics from your kitchen, food supply, water, and personal care products. Please review the chapter on toxins to refresh your memory about where these poisons are found and what to avoid.

Pesticides are in our homes, on our lawns, and on our foods. This requires you to become familiar with the Dirty Dozen and the Clean Fifteen lists so that you can choose organic products where the pesticide exposure potential is greatest. Of course, it would be best to eat totally organic products. Remember that pesticides are also hidden in the ingredients in the processed foods you eat. Look for alternatives to spraying pesticides in your home and on your lawn.

Pharmaceutical residues are a big concern. These include those produced from the manufacture of antibiotics, hormones, steroids, and chemotherapy agents. They are in the water we drink. Reverse osmosis water will remove most of them.

Herbicides like Atrazine and Glyphosate are in our water. Reverse osmosis will remove them. Try not to use them around your home and use alternative weed killers. Perchlorate (rocket fuel) is also in our water and must be removed as it is found in most of our bodies already. Fire retardants (PBDE's) are a big problem, present in the dust in your home, and can make you very sick, especially your children. Remove the dust with a HEPA vacuum.

Remember that heavy metals like lead, arsenic and mercury are in this category of Endocrine Disruptors. Lead is stored in bone and comes from old paints, drinking water, cosmetics and air pollution. Lead causes numerous serious health issues, especially in children. Arsenic is a deadly toxin and results in cancers and many other health problems. It is found in drinking water and US rice and rice products, grape juice and apple juice, which must be avoided. Mercury is in the air, oceans and lakes and can be released from dental amalgams. It concentrates in fish and you need to be aware of which fish are safe to eat and how much is a safe amount to consume. Use the Seafood Calculator from EWG to help. Remember, no canned tuna!

Triclosan is the main ingredient in antibacterial soaps, dishwashing liquids and other products. It is a potent Endocrine Disruptor and needs to be eliminated from your home. PFC's in non-stick cookware and on water resistant coatings are present in the bodies of 99% of our population. They never degrade in the environment and cause numerous serious health issues; they must be avoided. Solvents like glycol ethers are also Endocrine Disruptors and are present in paints, cleaning products, brake fluid and cosmetics. Nonylphenol results from the breakdown of nonionic surfactants in home and industrial uses. It contaminates our ground water, fresh water bodies, and fish. Look for these toxins and avoid exposure to them. We will look at detoxification for POP's later.

PFH Action Point

- POP's are Endocrine Disruptors and our environment is filled with them
- Plastics are everywhere and must be eliminated from your kitchen and personal care products
- Pesticides can be avoided by eating more organic produce and not spraying in your home
- Pharmaceutical residues and herbicides must be removed by reverse osmosis and fire retardants (BPDE's) by HEPA vacuuming
- Learn the sources of lead, arsenic and mercury to avoid exposure
- Triclosan, PFC's, solvents, and nonylphenol are other Endocrine Disruptors to be avoided

Volatile Organic Compounds (VOC's) are present in carpets, paints, particle board, adhesives and deodorizers. They cause very serious health problems. Try to avoid them and use air purifiers that are specifically rated to remove them. It is best to get rid of all carpeting in your home as it not only releases VOC's, but it retains pesticides and is a source of toxic mold. Start using VOC-free paints and cleaners. Get rid of room deodorizers as they are full of poisons.

Personal care products are loaded with Endocrine Disruptors and you need to be meticulous as you decide what goes on your body. Remember that your skin is the largest organ of your body and that these products are absorbed through it to lodge in your body and ruin your neurologic, endocrine and immune systems. These products include shampoos, conditioners, coloring agents, straightening agents, cosmetics, skin care products, sunscreens, baby powders and lotions. The toxins include phthalates, fragrances, dyes, heavy metals, and glycol ethers.

Remember that the average woman puts on over 16 different products every morning containing an average of 10 chemicals each; that is 160 chemicals every morning, many with known toxic effects. Women eat over 6 lbs. of lipstick in their lifetime, much of it containing lead. Out of the 85,000 registered chemicals, over 90% have never been tested for human health effects. Use the Skin Deep database to make healthier choices for personal care products for you and your family.

Electromagnetic Field (EMF) exposure is a real threat and I urge you to re-read the information I presented earlier. Electrosmog, as it is called, is not just cell phones and microwave towers. It includes low level radiation and very low frequency voltage (dirty electricity) exposure. It disrupts brain waves, causes behavioral and neurologic problems, allows the accumulation of Free Radicals, and damages DNA. Learn ways to prevent exposure and how to treat it.

Biotoxins are the next wave of knowledge that will hit the medical establishment. They result in Chronic Inflammatory Response Syndrome (CIRS) and an immune system that is chronically inflamed. This results in many illnesses, often masquerading and called something else, such as Fibromyalgia, Chronic Fatigue Syndrome, thyroid and adrenal disease, Autoimmune Disorders, Leaky Gut Syndrome, ADD/ADHD, Autism, Depression, and Unrelenting Fatigue.

The most common culprit in Biotoxin Illness is toxic mold from the interior of a water-damaged building (WDB). 50% of buildings in America are water damaged and potentially harbor toxic mold. Post Lyme Syndrome is another culprit. The incidences of Lyme disease is going up dramatically, with over 300,000 new cases reported per year. It is all based on genetics, with 24% of the population susceptible to toxic mold and 20% susceptible to Post Lyme Syndrome. The treatment is complex, but very effective. It needs to be performed by a physician familiar with Dr. Shoemaker's protocols at Survivingmold.com.

PFH Action Point

- **VOCs in our homes need to be eliminated; get rid of your carpet**
- **Personal Care Products are loaded with Endocrine Disruptors; use the Skin Deep database**
- **EMF is causing many health issues; avoiding it requires tough choices**
- **Biotoxins like toxic mold and Lyme Disease are often hidden and called something else; they require a careful search, elimination and treatment by a specialist**

Chapter 11
VITAMINS AND SUPPLEMENTS FOR HEALTH

Supplements are big business. Billions of dollars are spent each year on them. Some are very good, but many are not. If you open up a good supplement company magazine, or look online, you probably feel overwhelmed. All of the products sound great for your health and the companies are telling you that you must take all of them. Some are backed up by scientific research, but many are just people saying they feel better taking them (anecdotal evidence). What are we to do?

I use quite a few supplements in my practice. Remember, I am dealing with some very sick people. Their body systems are out of balance and they have numerous vitamin and nutritional deficiencies that I have documented through appropriate testing. Most healthy people don't need a ton of supplements, but some are of great help. My job as their Functional Medicine doctor is to advise them as to what is needed and what is optional. Some things are just a waste of money. I also try to guide patients toward reputable companies that have high quality standards for production of their supplements and do the research to prove that they are effective.

The standard medical and nutritionist response is that supplements are unnecessary and that you can get everything you need through your diet. This just does not stand up to what the current research is showing. Good studies are coming out regularly as to how supplementing with a certain nutrient decreases cancer or cardiovascular risk, increases life span, or improves the quality of life. The whole field of Anti-aging

Medicine seeks to help people age gracefully and often uses supplements as part of the regimen.

Traditional medicine seems to lag behind about ten years from what the research is saying about nutrients and supplements. For example, I remember the days when fish oil was only used by a few of us and the rest of the medical establishment was ignoring its benefits. What changed? A pharmaceutical company came out with a brand name prescription fish oil and did a lot of marketing. All of a sudden, it was now OK to tell people to use fish oil, especially if it was the prescription one. The same is true for CoQ10. It was ignored by the medical establishment and those recommending CoQ10 were labeled as unscientific and somehow ignoring the "standard of care". Now, cardiologists and others are recommending CoQ10 for specific conditions.

Look at Vitamin D. I remember when anyone recommending it was labeled as a nut. They claimed you could get plenty from drinking fortified milk. Then, there was the big admission that perhaps people were not getting enough because we were telling them not to drink milk. So, the RDA was placed at 400IU. Those of us in Functional Medicine were saying all along that this was inadequate and that we should be monitoring blood levels of D3. Vitamin D controls and impacts almost every organ system and metabolic pathway in your body. It is really a hormone and not a vitamin. Your immune system and thyroid are dependent upon having adequate levels. Then, the RDA was increased slightly to 800IU. We were using 10-20,000IU routinely to get blood levels up to a reasonable range. Now, there is a push to get the RDA up to 1200IU. That is still not enough.

Epidemiological studies now show that increasing Vitamin D3 levels above 30 will decrease a lot of diseases and prevents illness as the immune system functions better. There have been estimates of preventable deaths from low levels of D3, in the millions. While the medical establishment is lagging behind, people are dying needlessly from preventable illnesses and diseases. I use a blood level of 60 for my sick population of patients, but 50 is a good number for most people. Again, traditional medicine is behind the times.

Why does this happen? Physicians are trained in medical school, internship, residency and fellowship a certain way by a certain group of doctors. That way is grilled into them. When they are done, they usually continue treating patients the way they were taught. It can take a long time to change habits. Remember, the pharmaceutical companies usually run the continuing education programs, so there is a bias toward prescribing their medications as opposed to inexpensive supplements with less side effects. Again, it can take 10 years or more to change these habits even though the research is available documenting the effectiveness and safety of supplements.

I want to go over with you some basic information on supplements and make a few recommendations consistent with our goal of an **anti-inflammatory lifestyle**.

Why are vitamins and supplements needed? After all, God designed our environment so that we would be able to obtain everything we needed from the foods we eat and what we drink. So what happened? I believe that there are several reasons for this need for supplements.

The soil has been over-farmed and the land has not been replenished. This is a basic concept in farming that has been lost in our era of Big Ag and the need to make the most money by producing the most product. God told the nation of Israel to rest the land every 7 years for this very reason. The nutrients in the soil have been depleted and so the produce does not have the same nutritional content it once did. Studies done on organic produce confirm that nutrient levels are generally 25% higher than standard produce. Even organic produce does not contain the nutrients our produce did, say 100 years ago.

Take iodine for example. We have known for a long time that the area around the Great Lakes has soil that has no iodine in it. This area was known for having high numbers of people with thyroid goiters, or enlarged thyroid glands, and was termed the "Goiter Belt". Since people only ate the produce grown in their area, this did not affect any other part of the country. Now, however, we consume produce from multiple areas of our country and, in fact, from all over the world. When you go to the grocery store, the produce section is now truly an international marketplace. Many areas of the world now have soil that is iodine deficient due to over-farming and not replacing iodine in the soil. This is part of the reason for our thyroid disease epidemic here and in other countries.

Another reason for the need for supplements is toxin exposure. We have covered this in detail, but our exposure to numerous toxins disrupts our ability to absorb nutrients in our guts. Lack of good bacteria in our guts (Probiotics) is also an issue. The prevalence of Leaky Gut Syndrome and resultant malabsorption of nutrients is part of this problem. Toxins also interfere with the utilization of these nutrients in our bodies. Supplying extra nutrients can overcome this toxic interference. Toxins result in the production of Free Radicals that damage cells and DNA structure. Antioxidants neutralize these Free Radicals, but we are not getting enough of them. Taking extra in the form of a supplement can help.

Let us take a look at a specific problem requiring supplementation. Vitamin D is normally produced by your skin in response to exposure to sunlight. In the past, people were outdoors more, working and walking, so that Vitamin D production was higher in the summer and fall. This would help carry us through the winter months when Vitamin D production would be lower and help prevent illnesses. Now, we are not outside during the sunny part of the day due to work obligations or fear of skin cancer. If we are outside, we are covered in clothing or high SPF sunscreens. Add to that the toxins in our personal care products that we apply to our skin, which interfere with Vitamin D production, and you can see how Vitamin D deficiency has become a problem. Supplementing with Vitamin D becomes essential to your health.

PFH Action Point

- **Vitamins and supplements are big business; you need to have a good reason to use each product**
- **Stay with reputable companies to assure quality ingredients and good absorption**

- **Over farming of the soil has resulted in depletion of nutrients**
- **Toxins and lack of Probiotics affect absorption in the gut**
- **Vitamin D is needed due to poor sun exposure and toxins, resulting in a lack of production by the skin**

Generally, I recommend most people start with a good multivitamin. There are differences in the quality of multivitamins, both in terms of their ingredients and their ability to breakdown and be absorbed. I like multivitamins made out of plants, fruit and vegetable based, versus made from a long list of chemical additives. They generally have a high ORAC score. We covered ORAC in a prior chapter. It is a measure of the antioxidant activity of foods.

Vitamins have been found at the bottom of the tanks in water treatment plants, intact! Yes, that means they passed through the body without ever getting broken down and absorbed. This has to do with how they are compressed to make all those chemicals or nutrients into a little tablet. They may also have a wax coating or other covering to make them go down easier. You need to make sure the vitamins you take can break down and be absorbed. Generally, the better brands make sure of that. Cheaper vitamins may not do what you want. Vitamins coming out in your stool are a waste of money.

Most multivitamins have some Vitamin D added. You need to look at the ingredients and make sure it is Vitamin D3 (cholcalciferol) as this is the active form and does not require additional metabolic steps in your body to be made into it, like D2 does. Unfortunately, most multivitamins have very small amounts of Vitamin D3, from 400IU to 2000IU. Again, you should be guided by your blood test to know how much Vitamin D3 to take. A general rule is that 5000IU will raise your blood level 10 points. So, if your level is 25 and you want it to be 50 (remember 60 is better), then you will probably need 15,000IU per day. Toxicity is very rare and only with very high blood levels. Someday, we may be saying that a blood level of 80 is better!

Selenium is a trace mineral that is very important for your immune system and your thyroid to function properly. It has been farmed out of the soil and it is hard to get enough of it in our diet. Some nuts are a good source of Selenium. You should take a supplement with several forms of selenium daily, usually a small capsule, at a dose of 200-400 micrograms. The amount in most multivitamins is inadequate.

Vitamin C is a very basic antioxidant and well known, but it is still very powerful in its ability to neutralize Free Radicals. Most people take Vitamin C for a cold or before an airplane trip, but it should be a part of your basic routine supplements. For normal conditions, consider taking 2000 mg per day in divided doses since it does not stay in your body very long. Vitamin C with bioflavonoids may be absorbed better and stay in your body longer; that is what I recommend. When you feel like you are coming down with something, increase to 4000 mg or more per day. Loose stools are the only limit to maximum doses of Vitamin C.

Vitamin E is another basic, but very powerful antioxidant. There are different forms of Vitamin E. Typical vitamins contain alpha tocopherol, a less expensive form. However, the other forms may have even more significant antioxidant effects. Gamma tocopherol is very powerful and you should consider taking it if you want more antioxidant protection. The dose is 200-300 mg.

PFH Action Point

- **A basic supplement regimen includes a plant-based multivitamin**
- **Vitamin D3 is essential; get a blood test and get your level to at least 50**
- **Selenium, a trace mineral, is important at 200-400 micrograms per day**
- **Vitamin C is a good antioxidant; take 2000-4000 mg/day**
- **Vitamin E is a good antioxidant; use Gamma Tocopherol at 200-300 mg/day**

Most people recognize that Potassium is very important for heart and blood vessel health, as well as numerous other conditions. You can get Potassium from beans, fish, fruits and vegetables. The highest Potassium containing foods are white beans, dark leafy greens like spinach, sweet and white potatoes, dried apricots, squash, yogurt, salmon, avocado, white mushrooms and bananas. If you tend to run low Potassium levels, a supplement may be needed.

Did you know that Magnesium is just as important? Magnesium is an essential co-factor in many body processes, perhaps 300 different biochemical reactions. You can't make energy without it. Your thyroid won't work right without it. The list goes on. Magnesium deficiency is running rampant in our society due to soil depletion and consuming processed foods that are missing it. Many physicians check for Magnesium deficiency using a blood test measuring the serum level. This is very inaccurate. There is no relationship between the serum level and what is present inside your cells. A better test is an RBC Magnesium level, which reflects the amount inside your Red Blood Cells.

The top Magnesium containing foods include dark leafy greens like spinach, squash, pumpkin seeds, mackerel and some other fish, beans, lentils, whole grains, avocado, yogurt, bananas, dried fruits like figs and prunes, and dark chocolate.

Magnesium replacement through a supplement is a little tricky. Many Magnesium products are located in the cathartic aisle in the drug store. That is because they cause loose stools. Poorly absorbed Magnesium, like citrate and oxide, are common products. The best form is chelated Magnesium, meaning it is attached to an amino acid for better absorption. It seems the most readily utilized is Magnesium bis-glycinate or glycinate. It is not usually found in your drug store, but in a health food store or online. 200 mg twice daily will usually correct most deficiencies without causing loose stools.

Calcium is an essential nutrient for many of our body processes. Everyone thinks about bones, but actually Magnesium may be more important for bone health than Calcium. It is also important for teeth, muscles, nerves, and a variety of hormones and enzymes needed for life.

Calcium is obtained in our diet from many sources. Since milk and dairy products are off our list of foods that we can eat, we can get dietary Calcium in other ways. Dark leafy greens, like watercress and kale, are high in Calcium. So is cabbage and bok choy. Okra, broccoli, green snap beans, and almonds have a lot of Calcium. Sardines, anchovies and shrimp are also good sources. Coconut milk has good amounts of Calcium.

Taking a Calcium supplement may be a good idea if you are not getting enough in your diet or have certain medical conditions like Osteopenia or Osteoporosis. Again, the form of Calcium you take makes a big difference in absorption and utilization. Calcium carbonate and citrate, common forms in supplements, are not absorbed well and you have to take a lot of it (up to 1500 mg per day) to get the benefits you desire; this can result in side effects and other health problems. Calcium is a potent inducer of acid production in your stomach and can cause reflux and gastritis. The best form is Calcium Hydroxyapatit. The usual dose is 600 mg per day in divided doses; you may want more if you have Osteoporosis.

Iron deficiency is rampant in our country. Without Iron, many metabolic pathways will not work properly. In addition, anemia (low Red Blood Cell counts) may result and thyroid function is impaired. Fatigue is a common complaint of Iron deficient patients. Iron levels are typically measured through blood tests, but all of these are not created equal. The serum Iron level can look good and yet you can still be Iron deficient. Ferritin is the storage form of Iron and may be a more accurate reflection of your body stores of Iron. I often see very low Ferritin levels in my patients. Levels under 100 typically result in impaired thyroid function.

Replacing Iron is also a little tricky. We have already identified the top Iron containing foods in a previous chapter. In review, these include clams, oysters and mussels (if you like those). Seeds like pumpkin, sesame and sunflower have a lot of Iron. Liver is a good source of Iron, but I don't like it and usually don't recommend it since the Liver is the body's filter for all kinds of toxins. Dried apricots, sun-dried tomatoes, and blackstrap molasses are other good sources. Dark leafy greens, like spinach and kale, and meats like beef, shrimp and dark meat turkey have a decent amount of Iron. Beans, lentils, dried thyme and parsley, raw cocoa powder, and nuts like cashews, pine nuts and almonds round out the list.

It is always best to try to obtain Iron in a natural form. Due to poor absorption, you may need larger amounts. Concentrating Iron containing foods in Super Food drinks, juices and smoothies may be a viable option. Sometimes an Iron supplement is needed. In many states, Iron supplements are now a prescription item due to fears of adults and children overdosing. For non-prescription strength, a chelated Iron bis-glycinate seems to be absorbed better with less GI side effects, which include nausea, constipation, and bloating. Start at a low dose (18-25 mg) and gradually increase while monitoring Iron and Ferritin levels.

PFH Action Point

- **Potassium is an essential nutrient obtained from certain beans, fish, fruits, and vegetables**
- **Magnesium is an essential nutrient obtained from fruits, vegetables, seeds, beans, fish and dark chocolate**
- **Calcium is an essential nutrient obtained from vegetables, nuts and certain fish**
- **Iron deficiency is common and should be checked by blood testing serum Iron and Ferritin levels; know the top Iron containing foods**
- **If using supplements, I prefer chelated minerals like glycinate or bis-glycinate for better absorption of Magnesium and Iron; Hydroxyapatit is the better form of Calcium**

Let's talk about Mitochondrial support. A lot of research is coming out about how to support these energy-producing powerhouses in our cells. It seems that as we age, our Mitochondria deteriorate and stop producing ATP, the energy of life. They are subject to Free Radical attack and damage, toxins poison them, and they are affected by nutrient depletion. Mitochondria make energy by a process called the Krebs Cycle, which most of us learned in school and promptly forgot it because we do not use that information daily. However, knowing the Krebs Cycle helps us understand how to best support the continued efficient function of our Mitochondria.

All of the things we have discussed thus far will support Mitochondrial function. The **anti-inflammatory lifestyle** I have been advocating will help, including the right diet, clean water, eliminating toxins, neutralizing Free Radicals, and taking some basic supplements. However, there are specific supplements that will help those with what is being called Mitochondrial Dysfunction.

Coenzyme Q10 (CoQ10) is a popular supplement that has finally hit mainstream medicine as the research has clearly shown positive health effects for numerous conditions, including Congestive Heart Failure. Its ability to strengthen the heart has a lot to do with how it improves the production of ATP. Since the Heart utilizes a lot of energy, we would expect this organ to be positively affected. CoQ10 is a cofactor needed for the last step in energy production. It is depleted as we get older and by numerous other factors. Statin cholesterol-lowering drugs are well known to deplete the body of CoQ10. CoQ10 also functions as an antioxidant to protect the Mitchondria from Free Radical damage.

Not all CoQ10 is created equal and the source is very important. I would stick with a major company. Ubiquinone used to be the only choice for CoQ10, but now we have Ubiquinol available as a supplement and it is much more bio-available than Ubiquinone. You need less Ubiquinol to obtain the same blood levels as Ubiquinone. For most people, a supplement of 50-100 mg of Ubiquinol from a good company is adequate. Don't get cheap supplements!

Another cofactor in energy production is Pyrroloquinoline Quinone (PQQ). Like CoQ10, it is an essential last step in ATP production and is depleted as we get older and by numerous other factors we have discussed. It is also an antioxidant that protects the

Mitochondria from Free Radical damage. This supplement will become better known and popular in the next few years. If you take it as a supplement, get it from a reputable company; a dose of 10-20 mg daily is adequate for most of us.

Several other substances seem to have support roles in Mitochondrial function, as well. Acetyl L Carnitine is an important amino acid inside the Mitochondria and a dose of 250 mg daily provides good support. R-Lipoic Acid is an antioxidant that has important functions inside the cell to protect the Mitochondria and other organelles of the cell; 100 mg seems to be a good dose.

PFH Action Point

- **Mitochondria are the energy-producing powerhouses in our cells**
- **Mitochondrial Dysfunction is the result of many diseases, toxins, and nutrient deficiencies and is the underlying cause of many diseases**
- **Supporting the Mitochondria is critical; the right anti-inflammatory lifestyle will help**
- **Supplements like CoQ10, PQQ, Acetly L Carnitine, and R-Lipoic Acid can improve Mitochondrial function**

We have previously examined Omega 3 fatty acids in detail. Should the average person take a fish oil supplement? It depends on your diet. Remember, the goal is to have the optimum ratio of Omega 6:Omega 3 fatty acids, somewhere around 3:1. Since our diets in America contain an over-abundance of Omega 6 fatty acids, this ratio is often much higher than the optimum, reaching up to 20:1. Since this ratio affects the fat content of our cell membranes, the result is dysfunctional cells. This is particularly true in the Brain, where high ratios of Omega 6:Omega 3, and thus low levels of Omega 3, affect many aspects of Brain function. Is the answer then to just take more Omega 3?

This depends upon whom you listen to. There is a growing body of research that seems to indicate that too much of a good thing is not good. Too much Omega 3, especially in supplement forms, can have negative health consequences by disturbing this optimum ratio of fatty acids. The first thing we need to do is to clean up our diet and eliminate toxins from our bodies. Often this will restore the optimum ratio of fatty acids for our cells to function properly. If you don't like to eat fish, remember that there are other non-meat sources of Omega 3 (like hemp and flax) that are converted to Omega 3 in your bodies under the right conditions. Please go back and review that discussion on good fats.

If you feel the need to take an Omega 3 supplement, here are a few guidelines. I often prescribe high dose Omega 3 supplements to my Biotoxin patients as they are doing the detoxification protocol. It is also useful for elevated triglyceride levels, Brain dysfunction, and **inflammation** (i.e. joints). There is definitely a difference in quality that we need to address. Omega 3 supplements are predominantly made from very oily fish, such as anchovies, sardines, and mackerel. These are harvested from an ocean that is very polluted and these toxins are stored in the fat of these sea creatures.

It is important that these impurities and toxins are removed before you ingest fish oil, usually in a capsule or liquid. There is an International Fish Oil grading system from 1 to 5. You want a grade 5 fish oil supplement. These are carefully treated to remove toxins and impurities, usually through a process of molecular distillation. The better companies will advertise this and may even display their fish oil grade. Don't get cheap fish oil. You will belch it up and be poisoning yourself at the same time.

Some authorities and companies claim that Krill oil is better than fish oil. They point to a few small studies showing better absorption of Omega 3 due to the phospholipids in the Krill. This may be true, but I don't know for sure. There is not a good way to examine the amounts of EPA and DHA in Krill and compare it to fish oils. Thus, it is hard to know how much to recommend for people to take. Since I am using high doses of EPA and DHA, I must stick with fish oil. If you feel you need Omega 3 as a supplement, you will have to decide on your own which is the best form to take. As for amounts, that is best to discuss with your health care practitioner.

Probiotics are an essential part of any supplement regimen and I am sufficiently convinced of their value that I recommend them to everyone. When it comes to Probiotics, there are a lot of products on the market and a lot of hype. I remember when there were only two or three Probiotics available from the more reputable supplement companies. Now, pharmaceutical companies have gotten into the game and have done intense marketing to physicians to prescribe their products. The good news is that this has resulted in more choices and lower prices. It has also brought Probiotics out of the closet and subjected them to more scientific scrutiny. It is clear that they are not all made the same or have the same health effects.

A Probiotic is a beneficial bacteria that helps maintain the balance in your body. While they do populate the colon and help with digestion and absorption of nutrients, they also populate your lungs, sinuses, mouth, reproductive organs and other places in your body. Your stool is predominantly made up of dead or living bacteria. These beneficial bacteria help combat dangerous bacteria and other microorganisms, including Candida and other fungi. Thus, they are important for your Immune system to function properly. Probiotics may also serve functions like aiding in the production of certain vitamins.

Probiotics are needed because the populations of these beneficial bacteria are reduced due to our diet and toxin exposure. Poor quality diets, particularly those rich in processed carbohydrates (wheat and sugar, sodas, fast food, etc.) allow the overgrowth of yeast and diminish the number of these good bacteria. Antibiotics, present in much of the meat and dairy consumed, as well as prescribed in excess in our country, will destroy these organisms and allow the overgrowth of antibiotic-resistant bacteria. Toxins in the food chain will also kill these organisms, affect the motility of the gut, and promote fungal overgrowth. Anti-bacterial soaps, mouthwashes, bubble baths, and the use of steroid inhalers and nasal sprays will destroy the good organisms and allow the overgrowth of yeast in other body cavities.

Probiotics are usually found in a capsule and may need to be refrigerated, depending on the method of preservation and the type of organisms. It should be noted that refrigeration of Probiotics may help preserve the potency a little longer, but these organisms are designed to function in the human body at temperatures above 98 degrees. Thus, it is fine to leave them at room temperature if you will use them by the recommended date.

Recently, there has been an emphasis on incorporating Prebiotics either in the capsule or by taking a second supplement. These are compounds that stabilize and nourish the bacteria. It is good to consider a Probiotic that incorporates a Prebiotic or consider taking a second supplement. There is also much research coming out about the different strains of Probiotics and how they target specific organs and body cavities, creating targeted Probiotic therapy depending upon the need of the patient. You should consider this when selecting a Probiotic.

One of the things I try to do for my patients is to help them navigate the confusing world of supplements, including Probiotics, in order to select the most efficacious and cost-effective ones. There are many Probiotics on the market, but only a handful of companies can prove that their Probiotic can make it from your mouth to your intestinal tract without dying along the way. 50 billion organisms sound impressive unless they all die in your stomach. The method of preserving, encapsulating, and protecting the organisms is critical. You should thoroughly research the company, its methods, and the published studies they have done that document the effectiveness of their product.

PFH Action Point

- **Omega 3 fatty acids have numerous beneficial effects for those without an optimum ratio of omega 6:omega 3 from diet or for specific health concerns**

- **Choose a fish oil supplement that is grade 5 and molecularly distilled to remove toxins**
- **Probiotics are beneficial bacteria depleted in our bodies from poor diet, toxins, and antibiotic exposure**
- **Choose a Probiotic (combined with a Prebiotic) from a reputable company with published proof that it works and based upon the effect desired**

We talked about antioxidants in a previous chapter. If you recall, antioxidants are God's defense mechanism against Free Radicals. While we manufacture some in our bodies, such as Glutathione, which is the primary antioxidant within our cells, most of the antioxidants we need come from our diet. We need a broad spectrum of antioxidants to neutralize the five main Free Radicals in our bodies. When diet alone is not enough, then supplements are an option. Given the toxins we are exposed to on a daily basis, I highly recommend supplementing with antioxidants to protect our DNA and cells from oxidative damage.

The optimum source of antioxidants is a diet full of fresh fruits and vegetables. Remember that the antioxidant capacity of foods varies greatly and is affected by the time it takes to get from the field to your mouth, including time spent in the refrigerator. Antioxidant capacity is measured by the ORAC score, which we discussed at length previously. Make sure you are familiar with which foods have the highest ORAC scores so that you can focus on consuming more of them. Recall that raw, unprocessed Cacao is the highest antioxidant food on earth. God is so good that He made cocoa good for us!

A tasty way to get a variety of high antioxidant Super Foods is by making a Super Food smoothie. We discussed that in a previous chapter. Done properly, a smoothie full of Super Foods will supply your body with high quality protein, fiber, the right ratio of omega 6 to omega 3 fatty acids, vitamins, minerals, and antioxidants. Please go back and review the information on Super Food smoothies. (Chapter 7, Page107)

Besides basic antioxidants like Vitamins C and E, there are several others that have benefit. Recent studies reveal that Resveratrol is a powerful antioxidant. While it is mostly known for being the primary active substance in red grapes, it is interesting that Cacao has more Resveratrol than red grapes. Taking a concentrated supplement of about 250 mg when you can't ingest enough in your foods is a good plan. Quercitin is another powerful antioxidant with numerous studies demonstrating its benefits. Quercitin is found in Cacao, leafy greens like kale, red onions and some spices like dill and cilantro. Taken as a supplement, 250 mg is a good dose.

The primary antioxidant in your cells is Glutathione. It protects your cells from damage caused by Free Radicals. Your body makes Glutathione as part of your Methylation Pathway. We will look at that shortly. You can generate more Glutathione by taking a supplement of N-acetyl cysteine (NAC) if your Methylation Pathway is working properly. Glutathione is not absorbed well directly so it is better to give this precursor. I use NAC in many patients that are undergoing detoxification to protect their cells. A good dose is 500 mg once or twice daily.

PFH Action Point

- **Antioxidants neutralize Free Radicals and are obtained by eating fruits and vegetables**
- **Super Food smoothies are a great way to obtain a variety of antioxidants**
- **Raw, unprocessed Cacao is the highest antioxidant food in the world; cocoa is good for you!**
- **Resveratrol is a powerful antioxidant present naturally in red grapes and Cacao, but can be taken as a supplement**
- **Quercitin is a powerful antioxidant present in Cacao, red onions, and spices, but can be taken as a supplement**
- **Glutathione is made in your body to protect your cells; you can increase levels by taking NAC**

Turmeric is a spice receiving a lot of attention in the literature. The active compound in Turmeric that is most studied is called Curcumin. Several supplement companies have capsules containing highly concentrated Curcumin. This is a potent anti-inflammatory and is being studied by several cancer centers for its anti-cancer activity. Curcumin is also beneficial in those with highly inflamed immune systems, like my Biotoxin patients, to restore some of the balance to the system. I take Curcumin daily as part of my regimen and I highly recommend it.

We have already looked at cruciferous vegetables like broccoli, cauliflower, Brussel sprouts, and kale and their numerous health benefits. There are supplements available with highly concentrated extracts of these vegetables in a convenient capsule form. This is especially helpful if your diet is limited for a time or because of a lack of access to fresh vegetables.

Milk Thistle is technically an antioxidant, but this herb is most noted for its ability to help the Liver with detoxification. We will look at that later. Since our Liver is stressed daily with removing toxins from our bodies, protecting it with Milk Thistle makes a lot of sense. Get a purified and concentrated form from a reliable supplement company. The active ingredient is Silymarin and a dose of 600-900 mg daily should be adequate for most of us.

Methyl donors are compounds that donate methyl groups to the Liver to aid in detoxification pathways. We are all generally methyl group deficient due to dietary inadequacies and the excessive amount that must be used daily to detoxify our bodies. A good methyl donor is MSM, which you may commonly see associated with Glucosamine and Chondroitin for joint health and arthritis treatment. The amount of MSM present in these formulations is not a lot. You are better taking a separate supplement to increase the amount of MSM. It is a good Anti-inflammatory compound and will help different kinds of pain. It is very safe and a dose of 1000 mg twice daily is a good place to start. I know patients who take 5000 mg twice daily in order to keep their arthritis symptoms at manageable levels.

Another methyl donor is SAMe. This is a very popular medication prescribed by physicians in Europe, but has become a popular supplement here in America. The role of SAMe in the Methylation pathway will be examined in the next section. It has been studied and compared to antidepressants and has the same or superior results without the side effects. A common dose is 400 mg taken once daily.

Vitamin K is also receiving a lot of attention in the literature. We seem to all be deficient in Vitamin K, just like D3. Many know of this vitamin as an antidote to clotting disorders caused by excessive blood thinners like warfarin. Because of this, it has received a lot of negative publicity, alleged to cause blood clots. This is not true. It does help your blood to clot properly. It also acts as a potent anti-cancer agent, prevents heart disease by preventing the entry of calcium into your artery walls, and supports brain health (preventing dementia). Vitamin K2 also helps to build bone, working with Vitamin D3, and is a great help in Osteoporosis treatment.

Vitamin K is a fat soluble vitamin and consists of several forms. K1 is found in certain leafy greens and goes to the Liver to make your blood clot properly. Vitamin K2 is made by the bacteria in your gut (hence the need for lots of good Probiotic bacteria) and goes directly to organs other than the Liver for use. One supplement that I use combines Vitamin D3, K1 and K2, and iodine together in one capsule that is very convenient and contains the right quantities of these supplements for several conditions that I treat.

PFH Action Point

- **Curcumin, the active component of the spice Turmeric, is a good supplement for everyone to take**
- **Cruciferous vegetable extract is good for those not consuming enough of these very important plants**
- **Milk Thistle is an important herb antioxidant to assist the Liver in detoxification**

- **Methyl donors like MSM and SAMe assist the Liver in detoxification**
- **Vitamin K (K1 and K2) supplements are needed as we are all deficient and help prevent many diseases**

Iodine deficiency is a common problem and responsible for many diseases. I want to take a little time to review this topic with you due to its importance. Iodine is a halogen chemical, generally present in the soil around the world. However, certain areas have no iodine in the soil and many more have very little due to over-farming and not replacing it. Populations living in these iodine deficient areas often develop enlarged thyroid glands, called a goiter. The area around our Great Lakes in the US is part of this Goiter Belt. In order to prevent these goiters, governments attempt to supply iodine to the population by way of Iodized salt or supplements, which may help prevent some conditions of iodine deficiency, but not all of them.

Today, due to a salt phobia, most of us are not getting nearly enough iodine in our diet to prevent diseases. Leaving salt on the table will cause the iodine to sublimate and leave the salt to enter the atmosphere. Cooking also removes the iodine from salt. Sea salt contains a decent amount of iodine and is the preferred way to obtain it, other than eating sea weed or kelp. It should be noted that only certain types of sea weed, especially the kinds near Japan, contain a substantial amount of iodine. Processed foods are generally devoid of iodine.

Iodine deficiency is responsible for many diseases. We will look at how it affects the thyroid gland later. For now, know that thyroid hormone is made out of iodine; if you don't have enough, you can't make it. Low levels also affect the ability to make T4 (inactive thyroid hormone) into T3 (active thyroid hormone). Either way, the result is Hypothyroidism. There are numerous health consequences of being Hypothyroid and taking thyroid hormone may not fix the problems.

Populations with low iodine intake, such as the US, have increase rates of breast cancer and Fibrocystic breast disease. The Japanese, with one of the highest intakes of iodine in the world, had virtually no breast cancer or Fibrocystic breast disease until the western diet began to creep into their society and people began to eat less seaweed and other iodine containing foods. Once the Japanese move to the US, their cancer rates become what they are for the rest of us. Other consequences of iodine deficiency include cognitive impairment and psychological disorders (perhaps because of the Hypothyroidism) and an increased rate of stomach cancer.

The Japanese safely consume up to 13.8 mg of iodine daily (generally 3-6 mg). While there are no adverse health consequences of this amount of iodine in the diet, there are numerous benefits. The Japanese have very low rates of thyroid diseases. This amount is also protective against dysplasia (abnormal, precancerous cells), breast cancer, and reproductive cancers. The average American consumes less than 1 mg of iodine in their diet daily. Could this be the reason for all the thyroid diseases, breast cancers and other reproductive cancers in our country? I remember when I first started looking into iodine and I was shown a map, at a conference I attended, of all the areas in the world where there are very low levels of iodine in the soil. Then another map was superimposed on it of the highest rates of breast cancers in the world. Guess what? They are the same areas.

Iodine is also a natural detoxifier. It displaces toxins from the cells and frees them for excretion, including heavy metals. While this sounds good, it can be a problem. I discovered this the hard way. I started taking a large dose of iodine daily and got very ill. I discovered that my thyroid antibodies had gone sky high. I had created damage to my thyroid from Free Radicals as the toxins were released because I did not have enough antioxidants in my body to neutralize them. I learned a valuable lesson about detoxification. You have to have adequate antioxidants before you begin to mobilize toxins.

You can get an estimate of your iodine sufficiency by checking a blood test called Thyroglobulin. This is a protein that carries thyroid hormone and its production is dependent on iodine. It will give you an idea of how good your iodine levels have been for the past few weeks.

Low levels are indicative of iodine deficiency. There are no good blood tests to measure iodine directly. Spot urine iodine levels only show you what you have consumed in the last day.

Generally, I place most patients on a supplement of 1 mg of iodine since we are not getting enough in our diet. This is safe and will boost iodine levels so that thyroid hormone is made and detoxification will occur slowly. If a patient is very iodine deficient, I may place them on 6.25-12.5 mg per day. At these doses, monitoring is needed to ensure there are no side effects, although the Japanese regularly consume similar amounts without a problem. Higher does, although advocated by some, should not be taken unless a physician knowledgeable of iodine use is monitoring you carefully.

PFH Action Point

- **Iodine deficiency is common in the US and causes thyroid disease, breast and other cancers, and psychological disorders**
- **The Japanese consume a lot of iodine in sea weed and have low rates of these diseases**
- **Iodine is a natural detoxifier, but you must have adequate antioxidants in your body to prevent Free Radical damage**
- **A supplement of 1 mg daily is a good idea.**

We need to talk for a bit about Methylation defects. When I was first starting out in Functional Medicine, I did not have a clue what this was all about. A Nutritionist that taught me a lot, Carol, kept talking to me about this problem. I took a look at the pathway involved and it was so complicated that I just decided to let her take care of looking into it and fixing the problems. Carol died and went to be with the Lord and then I was forced to learn about this in order to properly care for my patients. If it was that important to her, then I decided it needed to be for me.

The Methylation pathway is one of the most important pathways in the human body. I have reproduced a diagram of it below from the internet:

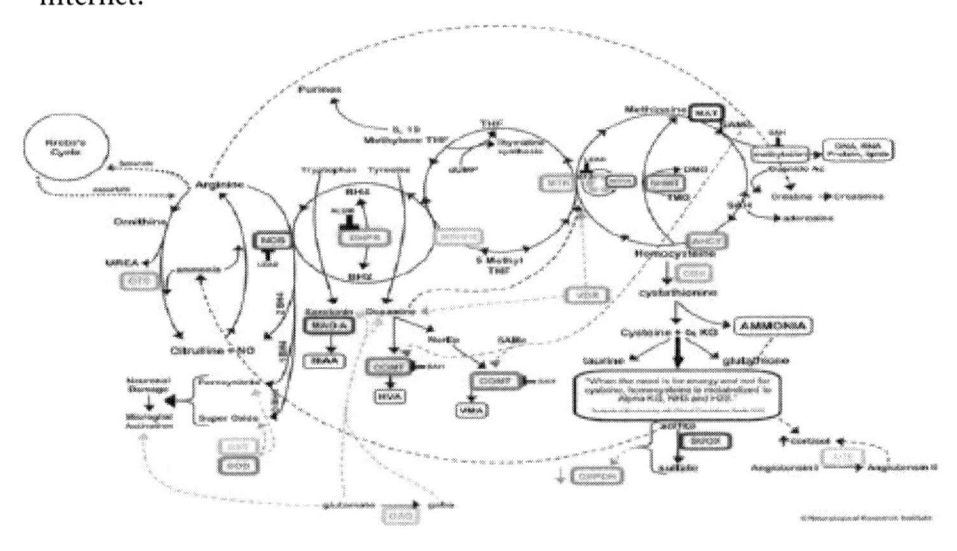

As you can see, there is a lot going on here. While I don't want to bore you or try to make you into a biochemist, there are some important take home points from this. Let me explain.

Methylation is important for several vital functions in our bodies. If you look at the right side of the diagram, you can see that one of the products of this pathway is SAMe, which aids in the repair of DNA, RNA, proteins and lipids that are damaged. Some people take SAMe as a supplement. This pathway is God's plan to prevent this damage and the resultant mutations from expressing themselves by way of the production of defective proteins and the growth of abnormal cells. The end result would be cancer. Cardiovascular Diseases like heart disease and stoke are also more likely. Other diseases associated with a defect in this pathway include blood clots, Autoimmune Disease (there are many of these), autism, migraines, Parkinson's Diseases, birth defects, psychological disorders (Alzheimer's Dementia, Schizophrenia, and Bipolar Illness), and Fibromyalgia/Chronic Fatigue Syndrome.

Further down the pathway on the right side, Glutathione is generated, which we discussed earlier and is the major antioxidant within your cells to protect them from Free Radical damage. Taurine is produced, which is a very important amino acid and helps to regulate brain chemicals, among other things. Sulfates are also produced which are needed during Liver detoxification pathways.

As you proceed to the left, the third circle involves the conversion of Tryptophan and Tyrosine to Serotonin and Dopamine. These important brain Neurotransmitters are essential to have in the right balance in order to think clearly and avoid depression and anxiety. The last circle on the left details the Urea cycle, which we will look at in a moment.

A clue that the Methylation Pathway is not working correctly is the production of excess Homocysteine. You will see this amino acid in the far right circle. This is easily measured in a blood test. Cardiologists recognize that elevated Homocysteine is a marker for those at risk from Heart Disease. They may not totally understand why that is, but now you will. Homocysteine is supposed to be in a steady state with Methionine. Both are amino acids. Methionine is obtained in your diet and those eating a lot of red meat will have higher Methionine levels and therefore may have higher Homocysteine levels. Otherwise, elevated Homocysteine is a marker for a malfunctioning Methylation Pathway. Different labs have different normal values for Homocysteine. Generally, I want to see levels under 10.

Why does this go wrong? To answer that, you need to look closely at the second circle. This is the Folate cycle. Folate is a B vitamin, so it is obtained in the diet. You don't make it. Tetrahydrofolate (THF) is typically obtained in your diet or a supplement. So, low levels of THF can cause the pathway to malfunction. An RBC Folate level can measure Folate. Serum Folate levels often show higher levels than what are present in the cells, so an RBC Folate level is better.

THF is not the active form of Folate. It must be converted to 5-Methyl THF. If you notice, there is an enzyme that does this called MTHFR; I will spare you the real name. There is a significant portion of the population that has genetic defects in this MTHFR enzyme and therefore has a reduced ability to convert THF to 5-Methyl THF. This is particularly true of Caucasian people of European descent. It is this form of Folate that drives the first cycle to reduce Homocysteine levels and convert it to other things. If you have reduced 5-Methyl THF levels, the pathway does not work right.

Vitamin B12 has a lesser, but important role in this process. B12 is called Cobalamin and is obtained in your diet or a supplement. It also must be converted to an active form to function optimally in the body; it is called Methylcobalamin. You can bypass this process by taking Methylcobalamin and the Methylation Pathway will function better. Methylcobalamin is available as a sublingual (under the tongue) lozenge that dissolves and is rapidly absorbed.

Common genetic defects in MTHFR are C677T and A1298. These can be detected by blood testing. If you have one copy of either mutation, your enzyme functions at about 60%. If you have two copies of one of the mutations, your enzyme only functions at 10-20%. If you have both genetic defects, you are likely to have very serious health consequences.

If you have an MTHFR defect and a high Homocysteine level with a normal RBC Folate, what can you do to lower the Homocysteine, assist the pathway to work optimally, and prevent disease? You can take a supplement of 5-Methyl THF and bypass the enzyme conversion. This supplement is not hard to find.

If you notice in the first circle, there is a direct way to convert Homocysteine back to Methionine utilizing a substance called TMG (TriMethylGlycine). This is a supplement that I frequently use to bring down levels not responding to 5-Methyl THF alone. Methylcobalamin (the active form of B12) is also good to take; it is in the form of a sublingual (SL) lozenge that melts. 5 mg twice daily is a good dose and makes B12 injections generally unnecessary. Check your serum B12 levels with a blood test.

If Homocysteine levels are very high, I will often prescribe SAMe to protect the cells and generate Methylation while we are working to reduce the levels. N-Acetyl Cysteine, which we discussed as a supplement precursor to make Glutathione, is a good idea to also protect the cells from Free Radicals, as Glutathione production will be depressed. For those with MTHFR defects, family members should be checked for Homocysteine levels and genetic testing done to avert damage from a defective pathway.

If you look at the entire pathway again, some things start to make sense now. If the Folate circle is not working right, then the Neurotransmitter circle does not work right, resulting in an imbalance of brain chemicals and cognitive dysfunction, such as Depression, Anxiety, Bipolar Illness, and others. The far left circle, the Urea Cycle, also does not work right and results in Free Radicals being generated and Oxidative Inflammatory Diseases. Do you see how important this pathway is to your health? You need to make sure your Methylation Pathway is working optimally.

PFH Action Point

- The Methylation Pathway is one of the most important in the human body
- Defects are suspected by elevated Homocysteine levels in blood and confirmed by genetic testing of the MTHFR enzyme
- The results of defective Methylation are cancer, Cardiovascular Diseases, and numerous other adverse health effects
- Treatment is to bypass the MTHFR enzyme in the Folate pathway and take 5-Methyl THF, directly lower Homocysteine with TMG, and take Methylcobalamin SL
- Have your Homocysteine level checked, along with B12 and RBC Folate. Do genetic testing if Homocysteine is high and RBC Folate normal

Leaky Gut Syndrome is a common disorder in our country and is known by many other names, including Irritable Bowel Syndrome (IBS), Functional Bowel, and Spastic Colon. In this disorder, the lining of the intestinal tract is inflamed and the absorption of nutrients is affected. I commonly see lower levels of Iron, Magnesium, B12, Zinc, and Folate in these patients. Proteins and good fats are also not absorbed well. Symptoms include diarrhea, constipation, or both; bloating; gut pain and spasms; and gas. There are often intolerances to many foods. For those with loose stools, urgency is a big problem and they must be near a bathroom after they eat. For those with constipation, having a bowel movement is a chore and often involves the use of laxatives.

Since your gut is a major part of your Immune System, there are consequences of it not working right. More frequent infections result and they don't resolve quickly. An overgrowth of Candida (yeast) is common in Leaky Gut patients, which worsens gut and Immune System problems. Lifestyle is affected, as the bathroom always needs to be available. For those with constipation, Diverticular Disease, bleeding and hemorrhoids are common.

Healing the Leaky Gut first involves dietary and lifestyle changes that we have discussed previously. All wheat and dairy must be eliminated, as these are frequent culprits in this disorder. Toxins must be avoided, including high fructose corn syrup, artificial sweeteners, GMO foods, pesticides and plastics. Sodas and coffee can aggravate this condition and must be avoided. Food allergy testing can be helpful to avoid foods that aggravate the **inflammation**.

As for supplements that can help, Probiotics are a must. We looked at those earlier. Get a good one made by a company that does the testing to insure it works. Slippery Elm Bark is a Native American remedy that has been used for centuries. It is very safe and very effective. It reduces the **inflammation** in the gut lining. Usually taken as a capsule several times daily, it has a healing effect on the gut. Aloe Vera juice is very soothing on the gut lining. Many Aloe products taste terrible, but George's Aloe does not. There is no maximum dose, but a good place to start is 2-3 ozs. twice daily. Glutamine is the most predominant amino acid in the intestinal tract and taking a supplement of it can help gut **inflammation**. Since Glutamine is a brain excitatory neurotransmitter, anxiety can limit its use in some people.

PFH Action Point

- **Leaky Gut Syndrome is a common disorder, often known as Irritable Bowel Syndrome (IBS)**
- **It results in diarrhea, constipation, and malabsorption of nutrients**
- **Lifestyle changes, including dietary modifications and eliminating toxins, are the place to start with treatment**
- **Several supplements can help, including probiotics, Slippery Elm Bark, Aloe Vera juice, and Glutamine**

Let us spend a few minutes discussing brain chemistry and natural supplements to help with anxiety and depression. As covered previously, anxiety and depression are two of the most common complaints to a family doctor and occupy top spots on any list of medications prescribed in our nation. Adopting an **anti-inflammatory lifestyle** helps balance brain chemicals and greatly decreases these symptoms. When that is not enough, then several natural supplements will help.

While brain chemistry is quite complicated, let me try to simplify it for purposes of this discussion. There are two major groups of brain chemicals. Excitatory neurotransmitters are designed to wake the brain up and get it ready for quick decisions and actions. Histamine, PEA, and Glutamate are examples of these chemicals. Inhibitory neurotransmitters are designed to calm the brain down and are often called "feel good" chemicals. These include Serotonin, Dopamine, and GABA. Normally, these chemicals should exist in a delicate balance based on the current needs. Imbalances are often the result of toxins, diet, medications, sleep dysfunction, and stress. When these imbalances persist, a diagnosis of anxiety or depression is sure to result.

According to <u>The Chemistry of Calm</u> by Dr. Henry Emmons, there are several natural supplements that can be used to manipulate these brain chemicals into a more favorable balance. A Psychiatrist with many years of experience, Dr. Emmons uses these supplements in his practice and they work well. I have used them in my practice for some time and can testify that they do work well for most patients and are fairly safe.

Theanine is an extract from Green Tea and has a profound effect on increasing GABA and Dopamine levels, both important to combat anxiety. 100-200 mg up to three times daily works well. Combining it with Lemon Balm seems to increase its effects. Tryptophan and 5-HTP are both final steps in the manufacture of Serotonin in the body and will increase its production. Remember that anti-depressant medications are usually blocking the re-uptake of Serotonin to leave it in the synapse longer. Eventually the body degrades it and, unless you manufacture more Serotonin, the levels will decline, requiring an increase in medication. Making more Serotonin makes a lot of sense. A dose of 500-1000 mg Tryptophan twice daily will work well.

Taurine is an amino acid that helps regulate the two types of neurotransmitters, specifically balancing Glutamate and GABA. 1000 mg twice daily is a good dose to decrease excess Glutamate. Rhodiola is an herb known as an Adaptagen because it assists the adrenal gland in adapting to stress by decreasing the production of the stress hormone Cortisol. Excess Cortisol can cause anxiety symptoms. 250 mg two or three times daily will help inappropriate rises in Cortisol levels.

Other helpful supplements include Inositol 500-1000 mg twice daily to help with anxiety and panic attacks. Vitamin B6 12 mg twice daily can increase GABA levels. Magnesium glycinate 100-200 mg twice daily can block excitatory toxicity. And N-acetyl cysteine (NAC) 300 mg twice daily will increase Glutathione levels to protect cells from Free Radical damage resulting from stress.

PFH Action Point

- **You can use natural supplements to combat anxiety and depression when lifestyle changes alone are not enough**
- **Theanine increases GABA and Dopamine levels, calming neurotransmitters**

- **Tryptophan and 5-HTP increase Serotonin production, a calming neurotransmitter**
- **Taurine helps to balance Glutamate and GABA, decreasing excitatory symptoms**
- **Rhodiola is an adrenal adaptagen that decreases Cortisol production**

Exercise is an important component of adopting an **anti-inflammatory lifestyle.** I am including it here as it seems to fit in with a discussion of supplements due to the numerous effects exercise has on human physiology and well-being. Exercise aids in pain control and improves the quality and duration of sleep. It improves energy levels and combats fatigue if done in the appropriate way and the right amounts. Exercise aids in weight loss and helps prevent Osteoporosis and bone loss as we age. It strengthens the Heart and causes the growth of new blood vessels. Exercise helps Brain function and prevents dementia.

The minimum amount of exercise is 15 minutes 4 times weekly. Daily exercise is a great idea, but it is not practical for many of us. Exercise can be as simple as a brisk walk or as complex as a training course. The general categories include Aerobic training, which involves the utilization of Oxygen by the muscles and other tissues. Flexibility exercises are important, as we tend to lose that as we sit around and as we do heavy work. This makes us more prone to injuries. Resistance exercises include light weights and exercise bands, designed to tone up muscles and improve bone structure. Strength training includes weight lifting and other variations to build muscle bulk.

For many of my patients who struggle with Fibromyalgia and Chronic Fatigue Syndrome, complex and lengthy regimens of exercise are counter-productive and not sustainable. Many patients who have not exercised in years or struggle with other health issues are limited in their exercise capacity. Just walking is a great start. Adding a recumbent exercise bike is another good choice. Water exercises have many benefits and are easier for many to do.

Doing exercise under the supervision of a physical therapist may be a good place to start if there are specific injuries or serious health concerns. A good personal trainer can help monitor and encourage you on your journey, as long as you set up goals and parameters with them and stick to them. Remember, it is more important to be consistent than to start an exercise program and quickly burn out. Find some things that you enjoy doing and stay motivated to do them.

PFH Action Point

- **Exercise is an important component of an anti-inflammatory lifestyle**
- **A minimum is 15 minutes 4 times weekly**
- **Walking is a good place to start; then progress to aerobic, flexibility, resistance and strength training as tolerated**
- **Exercise under the supervision of a Physical Therapist or Personal Trainer if you have health issues or injuries**

Chapter 12
SUPPORTING YOUR ENDOCRINE SYSTEM

As I began to dive into the world of Holistic Health and Functional Medicine, I quickly became aware of my need to learn more about proper functioning of our Endocrine system. Everything kept leading back to this. Poor functioning of the adrenal, thyroid, and hormone systems leads to many diseases and symptoms. These organs control most of what is going on in the human body. If we want to feel better and function at an optimal level, these Endocrine glands need to be in proper balance and performing the functions God created them to do.

I have to admit, it took a lot of work to review what I had forgotten about the Endocrine system and to learn all the new material that had come out. I discovered that there are really two different schools of thought on how to address this system. There is the Traditional Medicine view and there is the Functional Medicine view. Now, you would think that in medicine there would not be these vast differences in how to view and treat Endocrine disorders and imbalance. However, there are. Traditional Medicine looks with much skepticism on what Holistic practitioners are doing, despite current information in the literature and listening to what patients are saying about their experiences and how they feel. Things in Traditional Medicine change very slowly.

I decided to read, study and go to conferences in order to learn how to help people feel better, have proper balance, and decrease **inflammation**. This was over a decade ago. I experienced much ridicule during that time from other physicians specializing in Endocrinology. It is interesting to note that some of my Traditional Medicine colleagues have slowly gotten on board with this new point of view and are adopting some of these treatment principles into their practices.

While I don't intend to make you into an Endocrine specialist, as I am clearly not one, I would like to provide you with some practical information on a few very important parts of your Endocrine system. We will look at some physiology and discuss hormones and their roles in your body. We will look at imbalances that can occur and the symptoms that result. Finally, we will look at natural ways to support your Endocrine system. Remember, this is all an important part of our **anti-inflammatory lifestyle**.

PFH Action Point

- **Understanding and supporting the adrenal, thyroid and Hormone systems is very important to your health and healing**
- **Traditional medicine practitioners may not agree with our conclusions or therapy**

One of the first things I learned as I looked into Endocrine imbalances is that adrenal dysfunction is very common. I have to admit, I did not know a lot about the adrenal glands as most physicians learn those details in school and then quickly forget them. After all, we were told that adrenal diseases were uncommon. This could not be further from the truth.

The adrenal gland sits on top of each kidney and produces a host of hormones that regulate many aspects of your body. It is most known for Adrenaline, or Epinephrine, which is your "fight or flight" hormone. It helps you get in position to run fast or fight when threatened. This is only a small portion of what the adrenal gland makes.

The main hormone produced in the adrenal gland, from which all the others are made, is Pregnenolone. It is made from cholesterol. Don't let anyone tell you that cholesterol is bad. Small, dense LDL cholesterol may be bad because it has been oxidized. HDL cholesterol protects your blood vessel walls from oxidative damage by this small, dense LDL. Large, buoyant LDL cholesterol causes no damage and is being harmlessly carried through your blood vessels. Cholesterol is necessary for your body to produce hormones, especially in your adrenal glands. All the artificial lowering of cholesterol we have been doing in the past few decades with billions of dollars of medications coincides with the rise of adrenal dysfunction and hormone imbalances. Is there a connection?

While Pregnenolone has some independent effects, it is mainly important here because from Pregnenolone, two major hormones are produced by way of two different pathways. One pathway includes the production of Progesterone. After menopause, this is where most of the Progesterone in a woman's body is made since the ovaries have stopped producing hormones. Men are supposed to have a small amount of Progesterone also. Don't let anyone tell you that a low or zero Progesterone level after menopause is "normal" and a part of growing older for women. If so, why does every organ in a woman's body have Progesterone receptors? The adrenal glands are supposed to keep producing it. In many women and men, this does not occur due to adrenal dysfunction.

From Progesterone, the adrenal gland produces Cortisol and Aldosterone. Cortisol is your stress hormone. It aids the body to respond to physical and emotional stressors. We live in a society with more physical and emotional stress than any other in history. Continued excess production of Cortisol results in many deleterious effects, including central weight gain, high blood sugars, and vascular diseases. Eventually, Cortisol production begins to decline if continued high demands are made. Toxic interference also plays a major role in this decline. Examples are Biotoxins, which cause the disruption of a part of the brain called the Hypothalamus, responsible for generating a hormone signaling the production of Cortisol.

As Cortisol production fails to keep pace with the body's demands, a condition termed Adrenal Fatigue results. I treat many people with this condition. There are many symptoms, but the predominant one is fatigue, especially as the day progresses. A paradoxical awakening, a "second wind," often occurs between 10 pm and 1 am, resulting in sleep deprivation. Adrenal Fatigue patients often sleep best from 6-10 am. Adrenal Fatigue is confirmed using various blood tests to look at the adrenal hormones, as imbalances are the norm. Saliva testing of Cortisol levels at different times of the day will help to map out the patient's circadian rhythm, which now is not normal, confirming the dysfunction.

The other hormone made from Progesterone is Aldosterone. It controls salt and fluid balance in your body. When it is low, all kinds of problems can occur, including fluid retention, swelling, and Hypertension.

The other major hormone made from Pregnenolone, the other pathway in the adrenal gland, is DHEA. DHEA is a major hormone and recent research is confirming the necessity of having adequate blood levels of DHEA-Sulfate, the preferred form for measurement. Low DHEA-S is very common in my patients. Low levels are associated with numerous health problems, including immune system dysfunction, heart and vascular diseases, brain disorders and dementia, cancer and a general increased risk of premature death. Men have higher DHEA-S levels than women as it is technically an androgen, or male hormone. However, women need DHEA as much as men.

DHEA is converted to several other sex hormones in the adrenal gland. Again, if it is not working correctly, these won't be made. Testosterone is made from DHEA, especially in women. Women need some Testosterone, but not as much as a man. Again, it is made in the ovaries prior to menopause. It is made in the testicles in men prior to what is now being called andropause, or the decreased production of Testosterone as men get older. If the adrenal gland was working correctly, it would assume this production for men and women.

DHEA is also made into Estradiol, Estrone and Estriol. These three Estrogen compounds are very important in women's health. They are made in the ovaries prior to menopause. Men should have small amounts of Estradiol. If the adrenal gland is not working correctly, these hormones will not be made in adequate amounts.

It is interesting to conjecture that in the past, before our adrenal glands were under such an assault by physical and emotional stressors and toxic interference, adequate amounts of hormones were produced. Many women had no menopausal symptoms. Men remained virile and productive. God had this all worked out for us but things went awry.

Treatment of adrenal gland dysfunction includes many of the concepts we have already covered. You must have an **anti-inflammatory lifestyle**, including the right nutrition, adequate sleep, stress reduction, and elimination of toxins. Vitamins and supplements can be very helpful to restore proper balance. Exercise must be undertaken cautiously as too much can worsen the stress on the adrenal glands and further drive down Cortisol levels.

A useful supplement is an adaptagen like Rhodiola extract. It helps to modulate stress and allows the adrenal gland to rest, not producing so much Cortisol. 250 mg of a quality supplement two to three times daily is a common dose I use. DHEA replacement is something I frequently employ if levels of DHEA-S are not adequate. Again, obtain DHEA oral capsules from a reputable supplement company as they can vary greatly in potency. Consult your practitioner for the optimum dose. DHEA must be taken on an empty stomach to ensure adequate absorption and blood levels, usually one hour before breakfast or during the night if you get up. DHEA can also be added to topical hormone replacement prescriptions. Bio-Identical Hormone replacement may be needed if the hormone levels are not optimal. We will address that later.

PFH Action Point

- **Adrenal dysfunction is very common; it is due to physical and emotional stress and toxic interference**
- **Get to know the major adrenal hormones, such as Pregnenolone, Progesterone, Cortisol, Aldosterone, DHEA, Testosterone, and Estrogen**

- **Poor functioning of the adrenal gland is called Adrenal Fatigue and is very common**
- **Symptoms of Adrenal Fatigue include fatigue, sleep dysfunction, and hormone imbalances**

Thyroid disorders are nearly epidemic in the US. They are under diagnosed because of several factors. First, physicians rely very heavily on blood tests since they don't spend a lot of time talking to patients about their symptoms and lifestyle. The blood tests for thyroid disorders are flawed and have significant limitations, which we will look at shortly. Second, patients often put off being evaluated for their symptoms because they are too busy or just think it is normal to feel poorly, especially when it comes to fatigue and temperature problems. Many of us in Functional Medicine believe that the published figure of 7%, or 20 million Americans with thyroid problems, is greatly underestimating the problem. The figures may be closer to 30% of the population.

Many people with thyroid disorders are being misdiagnosed as having other problems. It is definitely a culprit in Fibromyalgia and Chronic Fatigue Syndrome, now called Systemic Exertion Intolerance Disease. It is well known that thyroid disorders cause Depression; how many of those people have been adequately tested for thyroid problems? Thyroid dysfunction also causes obesity, allergies, immune system dysfunction, heart failure, osteoporosis, cardiac rhythm disturbances, hormonal imbalances and gut problems like irritable bowel and constipation. Thyroid dysfunction may be a cause of cancer.

Thyroid controls your metabolism. It is essential for energy production, temperature regulation, immune function, bone growth, hormone balance, brain function and many other critical body processes. In order to understand thyroid better, we need to take a look at the production of thyroid hormone and how physicians use lab tests to detect and monitor thyroid function.

The thyroid gland sits at the base of the front of your neck and has two lobes, one on each side and connected in the middle. It is not easily felt and considerable skill and practice are required to detect subtle changes to it. Enlargement of the thyroid gland is called a goiter. Nodules can also develop, a small portion of which may represent thyroid cancer. With medication treatment, the thyroid usually shrinks down and is hardly felt, a condition we call atrophy. Autoimmune disease of the thyroid is unfortunately getting more common, a condition called autoimmune thyroiditis or Hashimoto's Thyroiditis; it can cause nodules or a goiter.

Thyroid hormone is made from combining four iodine molecules with an amino acid, Tyrosine; the result is called T4. T4 is basically an inactive form and is released into the bloodstream to be carried by a special protein to every cell in the body. Only the T4 that is in the "Free" form, not bound to proteins, can be utilized; this can be directly measured. Once at the cell, one of the iodine molecules is cleaved off the free T4 and Free T3 is formed, which can enter the cell and stimulate receptors affecting metabolism, etc. Again, only the unbound Free T3 is available to be used. This can also be directly measured.

A hormone from the brain, called Thyroid Stimulating Hormone (TSH) is released to tell the thyroid to make either more or less hormone. All major labs can directly measure TSH. It is released in response to T4 levels reaching the brain. It does not reflect the amount of Free T3 reaching the rest of the cells in the body. Therefore, using the TSH test alone can miss many Hypothyroid patients. I see this problem often.

There are many things that can go wrong in this process. Toxins, including the Goitrogens (chlorine, fluoride and bromine), interfere with the binding of iodine to Tyrosine and create under-production of T4. Nutrient deficiencies, particularly iodine and Tyrosine, also affect the production of T4 by the thyroid gland. Autoimmune disease gradually destroys the thyroid gland, affecting production, and can affect receptors for the thyroid hormone in the cells. These antibodies can be measured. The most frequently looked at is Thyroid Peroxidase Antibody or TPO. When there is not enough active thyroid hormone (Free T3) available for the body's needs, the diagnosis is Hypothyroidism. When there is too much Free T3 available and the body is over-stimulated, the diagnosis is Hyperthyroidism.

The conversion of T4 to T3 has many variables that can affect its efficiency. When it is poor, the term most often used is Functional Hypothyroidism. Poor T4 to T3 conversion is one of the more common conditions I treat and is often missed on lab testing and by most physicians. Remember, it is the amount of Free T3 getting into the cells and stimulating the receptors that is important for you to feel well, not the amount of TSH or Free T4. The factors affecting T4 to T3 conversion are many. I have to look for all of these when I treat patients with suspected thyroid problems.

The biggest factor affecting T4 to T3 conversion is the level of Cortisol from the adrenal gland. If it is too high or too low, the conversion changes. It has to be just right. The levels of DHEA-S, which we discussed above, are also very important; usually the problem is that the levels are too low. I was taught that you never attempt to fix the thyroid without making sure that adrenal function is optimal first. Over-stimulating the thyroid gland in a patient with adrenal fatigue will make them worse.

Autoimmune antibodies also affect T4 to T3 conversion, as well as damage the receptors within the cells. Nutrients are needed like iodine, Vitamin D3, iron, magnesium, zinc, copper, chromium, B vitamins and selenium. Low levels of any of these will decrease T4 to T3 conversion. Toxicity from exposure to Halogens (chlorine, fluoride, and bromine) will affect our conversion as well as our production of T4; that is why they are called Goitrogens. Birth control pills and oral estrogen medications will also affect this conversion.

Other factors affecting T4 to T3 conversion include ingestion of too much cruciferous vegetables and soy. While regular intake of cruciferous vegetables has many positive health benefits as we reviewed previously, too much of a good thing may not be good. Soy can be a problem from many perspectives, as we examined earlier, but here it is a problem by interfering with T4 to T3 conversion if taken in large amounts.

Toxins are major culprits in our decreased ability to convert T4 to T3. Tobacco, alcohol and caffeine all directly suppress this conversion. Endocrine Disruptors like plastics, pesticides, lead, mercury and other heavy metals, pharmaceuticals, food additives and preservatives, and other POP's interfere with conversion. Don't forget about the Mycotoxins in water damaged buildings and in our foods. Surgery, radiation treatments, liver and kidney diseases all affect conversion. Finally, medications affect the conversion of T4 to T3 including steroids, B-Blockers, SSRI's (depression meds), opiates (narcotics), Lithium, Dilantin, and iodinated contrast used for CT scans and other diagnostic tests. All of these must be considered when evaluating someone who is not feeling well and has poor conversion of T4 to T3.

Thyroid Hormone Resistance is another problem that can occur. This is sometimes called Functional Hypometabolism. This occurs when adequate Free T3 is available and gets into the cells, but cannot bind to the thyroid receptors to cause the desired results. There is either a block (or a toxic interference) or damage to the receptors. Patients will still feel like they are Hypothyroid; in other words they have the right symptoms but the lab tests look good. This is also a common problem I see.

Thyroid Hormone Resistance occurs from abnormal Cortisol levels, just as it did in the poor T4 to T3 conversion discussed above. It also can result from inadequate Vitamin D3 levels; remember, the normal values your doctor and the lab may be using are probably not optimal. Low iron levels are a big problem in Hypothyroid patients and interfere with receptor binding as well as cause poor conversion. Many patients do not feel well until they get their iron levels up. Unfortunately, this often involves taking a supplement.

Thyroid receptors inside the cell can be damaged by Free Radicals and thyroid antibodies, which are common problems. Thus, the Free Radicals must be neutralized and the causes corrected. This involves increased antioxidant consumption. There can also be competitive binding at the receptors involving the Halogens, Mycotoxins and Endocrine Disruptors discussed above. As you can see, a lot can go wrong with the production and utilization of thyroid hormone. The process to search out the causes involves being a medical detective.

If you or someone you know has been diagnosed with Autoimmune Thyroiditis (Hashimoto's), don't be content with the answer that the antibodies are just there and won't ever go away and won't do anything bad. Wrong! It is not normal to have antibodies to your own thyroid gland. I had Autoimmune Thyroiditis with antibody levels in the thousands. I have had no antibodies for years now. The underlying problem can be corrected and the antibodies go away. This involves meticulous attention to diet and increasing antioxidant consumption both in foods and in supplements. Toxins must be eliminated. It goes without saying that if you smoke or drink, it will never go away. Elimination of wheat, dairy, HFCS, GMO's, artificial sweeteners, MSG and other food additives, Nitrites and other food preservatives, and mycotoxins is essential. The gut must be healed and any Methylation defects corrected. iodine replacement is very important if levels are low.

If the production of T4 is impaired after correcting the nutrient and toxin variables we have just covered, thyroid hormone supplementation is probably needed for the patient to feel well. Again, this will not work if there is decreased conversion of T4 to T3 or the receptors in the cells are either blocked or damaged. Those things must be corrected. Several options are available by prescription for thyroid hormone. They must be started at a low dose and carefully increased under close monitoring.

Levothyroxine (Synthroid) is T4 made in a laboratory. Many patients do not feel better on Synthroid because the other factors have not been corrected and they either can't make it efficiently into Free T3 or can't get it to work properly in the cells. The generic Levothyroxine has had many quality problems and it is best to get the real Synthroid. It is the preferred option if there is Autoimmune Thyroiditis present because patients with that disorder tend to get worse on Porcine Thyroid.

Porcine Thyroid (Armour, Nature) is made from pigs' thyroid glands and is purified and standardized by pharmaceutical companies. The advantage is that it contains T4, T3, Calcitonin and other thyroid hormones and nutrients; the medications contain the basic raw materials the thyroid needs and patients often feel much better on them. T3 is available as a pharmaceutical (Cytomel). It is useful short term to get T3 levels up when patients are not converting properly and we are waiting for the detoxification to be completed. Compounding pharmacies can make pure T4 and T3 in any combination and without some of the fillers that patients can react to.

PFH Action Point

- **Thyroid disorders are epidemic in the US and include decreased production, poor T4 to T3 conversion, thyroid receptor problems, Autoimmune Thyroiditis, and Hyperthyroidism**
- **There are limitations to the commonly used thyroid blood tests; TSH often misses the diagnosis; Free T4 and Free T3 levels are better measures**
- **There are many nutritional deficiencies and toxins that can interfere with thyroid function**
- **It is important to correct adrenal dysfunction before taking thyroid medication**

A thorough discussion of hormone balancing is beyond the scope of this book. It takes me a lot of time to evaluate all of the factors that go into balancing hormones for men and women. It is not just as simple as writing a prescription for hormones. However, there is some information that I believe is important for you to have.

For the purpose of this discussion, when I refer to hormones, I will mean the sex hormones. These include Progesterone, Estrogen compounds, DHEA and Testosterone. Prior to menopause (and andropause for men), these hormones are primarily made in the ovaries and testicles. After menopause and andropause, they are made in the adrenal gland. There are many factors influencing deficiencies or excesses in hormones. We have already covered many of them. These include nutritional deficiencies, toxins such as Endocrine Disruptors, sleep dysfunction, stress, medications and exercise. As we adopt our **anti-inflammatory lifestyle**, we can fix many of these hormone imbalances.

As we discussed above, adrenal and thyroid disorders directly impact hormone levels. Only when these factors are corrected should we consider Hormone Replacement Therapy (HRT). I see this as a frequent problem in new patients. They have symptoms of hormone imbalance and are on hormone therapy. As we talk more, it is obvious that the patient is not pursuing the right nutrition, toxin elimination, and the other essential parts of our **anti-inflammatory lifestyle**. Their adrenal and thyroid function has not been adequately balanced. They want more hormones. Do you see the faulty logic? If a little is good, a lot must be better. This only results in serious and unwanted side effects.

Symptoms of hormone imbalance include fatigue, mental fog, bone loss and Osteoporosis, muscle loss, weight gain, and depression. You can see how these overlap with several other conditions we have discussed, including thyroid and adrenal disorders, Biotoxin Illness and Mycotoxins exposure, and toxicity by Endocrine Disruptors. These must be addressed first. Remember that there are receptors for these hormones in every organ of the body. They must be important for our health overall, not just for sexual function. Vasomotor symptoms like hot flashes are particularly bothersome to women. I often have men accompany a woman for their visit and they beg me to give the patient hormones so that she will stop being a raving lunatic at times.

It is important to do the proper testing to diagnose hormone imbalances. The textbook that is used to train all residents in Obstetrics and Gynecology about Endocrinology states that there is no relationship between blood levels of hormones and tissue levels. Why do we do blood testing for hormones then? It is easy and insurance covers it. But blood tests are not accurate, especially for monitoring therapy. As we discussed in the thyroid section, it is only the unbound free hormones that are available to be used by the tissues of the body. Blood tests look at total hormone levels. They do not reflect tissue levels. Major labs do offer free hormone levels and these may more closely approximate tissue levels.

Make sure you are doing the right testing is you suspect a hormone imbalance.

A better method for testing hormones is saliva. We can assume the Salivary gland is an end organ and the concentration of the hormones in that organ will be the same as other tissues in the body. Saliva can be collected and measured for hormone levels easily, but be careful of the methods used by different companies, as they do not produce the same results. The hormones measured will be the free hormones, but may not be equal to those measured in the blood. Saliva testing is easy, inexpensive and very accurate. Once you are on topical hormone therapy, this is the only reliable way to measure tissue hormone levels and monitor therapy.

Once a decision is made to prescribe hormone therapy, either temporarily or more permanently, a decision needs to be made as to the route of delivery. While pills are more convenient, they are not optimal and do not produce consistent tissue levels. The liver takes out a lot of the hormones from your system and they are never utilized. This can vary from day to day. Topical therapy is much better, either in a cream, gel or patch. It produces fairly consistent tissue levels if applied properly. We can also utilize sublingual lozenges (under the tongue) for rapid absorption into the blood when topical treatment is not appropriate.

The type of hormone used is critically important. This discussion concerns the differences between pharmaceutical company hormones and Bio-identical hormones. You will hear and read a lot of rhetoric about this topic. As a holistic practitioner, I did a lot of my own investigation into this topic to insure that my patients were getting the most efficacious and safest treatment. After a thorough review, I concluded that Bio-identical hormones were safer and provided better results. Compounding pharmacies are particularly knowledgeable about these hormones and the various methods of application. Many experienced pharmacists are good at troubleshooting problems that can occur with patients on hormones. Seek out a good compounding pharmacy and find out from them who is a good local practitioner who knows what they are doing with balancing hormones naturally.

One last thing about hormone therapy that does impact our **anti-inflammatory lifestyle**. Hormones can become a toxin if dosed too high. Why would this happen? Again, patients can assume that if a little is good, then a lot is better and can increase their own dosing to unsafe levels. You can absorb hormones from your mate, or at a gym off of the equipment if you are not careful, and develop high levels. Monitoring hormone therapy by blood testing instead of saliva testing can result in inaccurate hormone measurements and an increase in the dosing in response to symptoms. Failure to consider the way hormones work can result in super high dosing. Many offices will tell patients that call with bothersome symptoms that their hormones are too low and then increase them over the phone. This is generally a bad idea.

Hormones operate like a bell-shaped curve. When the hormones are too low, then you will have symptoms. When the hormones are dosed optimally at the peak of the bell curve, symptoms will be controlled as long as the other factors we have identified have been corrected (i.e. adrenal, thyroid dysfunction). When the hormones are dosed too high and the levels are now past the peak and coming down the other side of the curve, symptoms return and may be exactly the same as when the levels were too low. The response will be to increase the hormones, which will further aggravate the situation. This is when unwanted side effects may occur, such as the development of cancer. While cancer risk is much higher with pharmaceutical hormones, due to the way they have been altered to patent them, it is nonetheless present with all hormones prescribed at too high a dose. Seek to use hormones only within the therapeutic range recognized by a reputable saliva testing lab and experienced practitioners.

PFH Action Point

- **Balancing hormones should be done only after implementing our anti-inflammatory lifestyle and correcting any adrenal and thyroid dysfunction**

- Balancing hormones needs to be done in a cooperative fashion between you, an experienced practitioner, and a reputable saliva testing lab
- Using Bio-identical hormones is less likely to result in serious side effects than pharmaceutical hormones when monitored carefully
- Remember that if a little is good, a lot is not better

Chapter 13
DETOXIFICATION MADE SIMPLE?

I chose the title of this chapter as a question for a reason. I am not sure that the subject of detoxification can ever be made into a simple presentation. By its very nature, it is extremely complicated. I generally do a pretty good job of explaining complex things to my patients in simple terms that they can understand. I am not sure if I can do that here, but I will certainly try.

We have always been exposed to toxins. There have always been heavy metals such as lead, arsenic and mercury in our environment. God designed our bodies with an intricate, complex mechanism to remove these toxins and render them harmless, to preserve our health. Fortunately, these pathways are very efficient and can remove even toxins we are exposed to in our environment today that are not natural. Our detoxification (detox) pathways can handle metabolic end products, heavy metals, pollutants, toxins from microorganisms, alcohol and plant toxins.

Our systems have been overwhelmed by the quantity of toxins we are exposed to since the advent of the industrial age. For example, studies done on the bones of deceased people show that bone lead levels have increased 1000 times since the industrial age began. The amount of lead and other heavy metals we are exposed to has overwhelmed our detoxification pathways. This is true of other pollutants, as well. Endocrine Disruptors and other man-made toxins have confused the detoxification pathways and occupy them excessively, not allowing them to work on other toxins. Pharmaceuticals and nutrient deficiencies have affected the Liver, its enzymes needed for detoxification, and other parts of the pathways.

Let me try to explain Metabolic Detoxification to you. I will try to make it as simple as I can, but this is a complicated subject. If you are not that interested in the physiology, you can skip parts of this section. However, try to absorb most of it so that when we discuss detoxification strategies for your health they will make more sense to you.

Metabolic Detoxification is divided into phases. Phase 1 involves the enzymes in the Liver transforming lipid-soluble compounds (those dissolved in fat) into water-soluble compounds (able to dissolve in water). The enzymes are predominantly called the Cytochrome P450 enzymes. This is important to make toxins available to be excreted by the kidneys later.

Phase 2 involves making the toxins less of a threat by conjugating them (attaching them) to other substances. This makes them less mutagenic and carcinogenic, or less of a threat to cause DNA damage and cancer. This process is under the control of NrF2, a master regulator of antioxidant response within the cells. This regulation will be important later. NrF2 senses oxidative stress and the presence of toxins (by phase 1 activation) and turns on the antioxidant proteins.

Phase 3 involves moving these enzymatic products out of the cells, by special ATP dependent transporters, for excretion from the body. They may be moved from the Liver into the bile, from the blood into the Kidneys, or from the Intestines back into the Intestines.

I hope it is obvious to all of you that this complex, inter-dependent system could not have just happened. To think, as I used to when I was an atheist, that this all just came about by way of random chance mutations over millions of years, is absurd. Every watch has a watchmaker. Our bodies have a Creator Who designed us with incredible complexity and beauty to function as it does.

PFH Action Point

- **We have always been exposed to toxins, even heavy metals**
- **Our systems have now been overwhelmed with man-made toxins they were not designed to deal with**
- **God has designed out bodies with an intricate, complex mechanism to remove toxins and prevent disease, but it has been damaged in many ways**
- **Metabolic Detoxification involves 3 Phases that you should try to know**

Knowing these detox pathways, let us look at some general things we can do to enhance detoxification by our bodies. This needs to be a routine part of your **anti-inflammatory lifestyle**. The most important thing is to begin to eliminate sources of toxins so that your detox pathways can keep up. This includes meticulously identifying toxins in your food, water, air, home, cleaners and personal care products and avoiding or removing them. The first part of this book was designed to help you do that.

Flushing with clean water is a critical part of any detox plan. Many toxins will be excreted by way of your kidneys. The detox pathways do not work optimally if you are dehydrated. Remember that you need either distilled or reverse osmosis water and that you should drink at least half your body weight in ounces each day. You need to drink out of glass or stainless steel containers and get rid of all the plastic water bottles.

An alkaline diet is also important, as an alkaline environment is needed for your detox enzymes to function best. An acidic diet results in your kidneys stealing calcium from your bones to neutralize your pH. An alkaline diet is best obtained by eating mostly fruits and vegetables, preferable raw or lightly steamed, and eliminating processed foods, wheat and sugar.

Exercise and sweating does remove some toxins. In fact, a sauna can be very beneficial. Studies show that sauna sweating can remove Arsenic, Cadmium, and some POP's.

Colon care is critical since many toxins will be eliminated in your stool. It is important to eat a lot of fiber, much more than you think you need and the government is telling you. With that, a lot of water is needed to hydrate the fiber. A good Probiotic is essential due to the depletion of our good intestinal bacteria by antibiotics and toxins. Aloe Vera juice can nourish the lining of your colon and revive it. Slippery Elm Bark is very healing for your colon lining. It is important to have at least one bowel movement daily. Magnesium and prunes can help with that. If you are hopelessly constipated, then you probably have other issues that need to be evaluated.

There are some general detox methods you may want to try. Drinking a glass of water with 1 whole lemon squeezed into it in the morning can rid your body of several toxins. Some advocate oil pulling. This involves holding one tablespoon of coconut or sesame oil in your mouth for 15 minutes in the morning. It is claimed that this oil will pull toxins from your body through the lining of your mouth and then you spit it out. While I have no controlled studies to prove this happens, it makes some sense if you can stand the taste.

PFH Action Point

- **There are general things you can do to enhance detoxification**
- **The most important is to try to eliminate ongoing sources of exposure to toxins**
- **Flush with clean water and consume an alkaline diet**
- **Exercise, sweating, use of a sauna, and colon care are important**
- **Water with lemon and oil pulling can be helpful adjuncts**

What can you do to enhance your detox pathways? Let's start with preventing absorption of toxins. Probiotics can certainly help with this.

Charcoal is well known to prevent absorption and I used it frequently in the Emergency Department to treat patients who had accidental or intentional overdoses of medications or other substances. Using Charcoal occasionally may be a good idea, but regular use may cause a lot of issues with your gut and prevention of nutrient absorption.

Some advocate the use of clay, including Bentonite clay, to prevent toxin absorption. Bentonite clay has a strong negative charge and contains an abundance of minerals. As it comes in contact with water in the gut, it is activated and attracts positively charged toxins, releasing its minerals for use by the body. Since Mycotoxins are negatively charged, as are many plastics and pesticides, it will not be effective for them. However, heavy metals are positively charged and may absorb them. Again, I don't have any personal experience and there are no controlled studies to demonstrate its effectiveness. I see no harm in its use. Chlorophyllin is another substance to prevent toxins from being absorbed; it has been especially looked at in regards to preventing Mycotoxins like Aflatoxin from being absorbed into the body. It is made from Chlorophyll, the green plant pigment, and is a potent antioxidant, protecting DNA from Free Radical damage.

Another way to enhance detox is to optimize bile secretion from the liver. This can be accomplished by using the following herbs and foods: artichoke, ginger, cumin, garlic, curry, dandelion, Yarrow Fennel and Andrographis. Try to incorporate more of them in your diet. Liver support can include the use of green tea, pomegranate, cruciferous vegetables, citrus fruits, watercress, and turmeric. Colon support is essential to enhance detox; see my discussion above.

Detox cannot proceed effectively unless Methylation is working optimally. We have discussed the Methylation pathway earlier in this book. If Homocysteine is elevated, or there is other evidence of impaired Methylation, it must be corrected or SAMe, Glutathione, and parts of the Liver detox pathway will not be optimally produced. SAMe aids in the repair of damaged DNA. Glutathione is the major intracellular antioxidant and must be present in adequate amounts to protect the cells and your DNA from Free Radical damage.

Inadequate iron levels must be corrected to enhance the body's ability to detox. When iron levels are low, the transport proteins in the gut and brain work harder to capture and absorb more iron. Unfortunately, these same transport proteins will capture and absorb more toxins, as well. This is not our objective. Iron levels need to be normalized. We have previously discussed iron containing foods and supplements to help.

PFH Action Point

- **You can enhance detox by preventing absorption of toxins**
- **It is good to optimize bile secretion and support the Liver**
- **Correct any Methylation defects or detox will not proceed effectively**
- **Correct any iron deficiency or you will absorb more toxins**

Let us look now at some specific nutrients that will enhance detoxification and how they affect the system. B Vitamins are essential for many of the enzyme reactions involved in detox. These come in your diet, but a quality multivitamin supplement is recommended for most of us, preferable plant based. Antioxidants are needed to protect your cells and DNA from Free Radical damage due to the presence of toxins in the cells and as toxins are released to be moved to the Liver. These include N-Acetyl Cysteine (NAC), which regenerates Glutathione, Vitamin C, Vitamin E (mixed tocopherols, including gamma tocopherol), cold processed Cacao, Resveratrol, and Quercitin.

Antioxidants are also needed to help activate NrF2. Remember, this is the master regulator of antioxidant response in the cells by sensing antioxidant stress and turning on the antioxidant proteins in the cells. Stimulating this response is a very good thing to enhance detox and protect the cells. Antioxidants that are NrF2 activators include Flavonoids (like Cacao), green tea, Quercitin, and Resveratrol. Super Food Smoothies are a great way to obtain all of these antioxidants.

Other NrF2 activators include turmeric (active ingredient is Curcumin), Tocopherols, Garlic, Gingko Biloba, and Chlorophyllin.

You can enhance detox by supplying more sulfur compounds for your liver to use in detox. Cruciferous vegetables and Indole-3-carbinol are great sources of sulfur and will also activate NrF2. Their added benefit is that they detoxify excess body estrogens, such as are found in Endocrine Disruptors. Citrus contains a compound called D-limonene, which is useful for chemoprevention (or chemoprophylaxis), the process of administering a compound to prevent disease. Sulfur compounds are also chemoprevention agents.

Mushrooms are helpful to enhance detox by supporting immune function. Of particular benefit are Chaga and Reishi mushrooms. I am allergic to mushrooms, so I can't eat these. If you are not allergic to mushrooms, then these would be a great addition to your nutritional program.

Let us look at some other substances and supplements that can enhance detox. We have already mentioned N-Acetyl Cysteine (NAC), which regenerates Glutathione. NAC is also a Free Radical scavenger on its own. It will bind to Methyl Mercury to excrete it in your urine. Selenium works with Glutathione as an antioxidant and will also bind mercury. Since we all have exposure to mercury in our foods and the environment, these are great supplements to take. Milk Thistle (the active ingredient is Silymarin) works by preserving Glutathione and acting as an antioxidant for your liver; thus, it is often mentioned as a part of liver support and is worth taking daily.

The detox pathways require Calcium, Zinc and Copper, so it is important to have an adequate supply of these nutrients. Remember that iodine is a natural detoxifier and will mobilize toxins from your tissues. As we discussed previously, it is important to make sure you have adequate antioxidant defense while you use iodine or the Free Radicals will cause damage.

You can take SAMe as a supplement to support Methylation and detoxification. Besides its role in DNA and RNA repair, SAMe acts as a methyl donor and aids the liver in detoxification. Most of us are not donating enough methyl groups to our Liver for detoxification. Taking a supplement like SAMe or MSM can help greatly.

There are specific detoxification protocols to follow when certain toxins overwhelm your system.

We have already covered Biotoxins like Mycotoxins and the organism that causes Lyme Disease. They require a very complex protocol to remove the toxin from your body and repair the chronically inflamed immune system. However, optimizing the entire detox pathway helps tremendously as all of us have numerous toxins we need to deal with simultaneously. Endocrine Disruptors such as the Persistent Organic Pollutants (POP's) also require specific detox procedures. Heavy metals that do not clear with the natural approach we are discussing will need more advanced measures such as oral, rectal or IV chelation. It is best to consult an experienced practitioner who specializes in these types of detox protocols and can closely monitor you.

PFH Action Point

- **Detox can be enhanced with the right nutrients, such as antioxidants to protect the cells from Free Radicals and to stimulate NrF2**
- **Sulfur compounds, like cruciferous vegetables, and mushrooms can enhance detox**
- **There are numerous supplements that can aid our detox pathways including Milk Thistle, iodine, and SAMe**
- **NAC regenerates Glutathione; together with Selenium, they bind mercury**
- **Specific toxins, such as Biotoxins, Endocrine Disruptors, and heavy metals, require more advanced detox protocols that need to be administered by an experienced practitioner**

Chapter 14
THE FINAL KEY TO HOLISTIC HEALTH

The goal that I have had in writing **Prescription for Health** has been to help you heal holistically: body, mind, and spirit. We have spent a lot of time on physical health and healing. We have discussed the need for emotional health and healing in previous chapters. When that is not possible on your own, God has created counselors and therapists who can try to help us.

Good counselors and therapists understand that real healing comes from the Lord. Only He is able to pull out the pains of your past, heal you of them, and help you to rise above them. There are many techniques available. If you can't defeat depression, anxiety, addictions to food and substances, fears and phobias, or a spiritual crisis, then you need to admit you need help and get it. Start with your pastor if you attend a church; if he or she can't handle your issues, they can refer you to someone who can. You can also seek out a Christian Mental Health professional or Christian Counselor.

Let's talk about your spiritual health for a few minutes. Why should we address our spiritual condition? After all, that is totally separate from my physical health, right? Sure, I will eventually get to my spiritual life someday. Right now, I have too much else to do and a lot to worry about. It's just not a priority in my life right now.

Perhaps you need to re-think that approach. My experience is that your spiritual health is every bit as important as your physical and emotional health. In many ways, your spiritual condition affects all of the other areas and your approach to life and health. I have witnessed this in my Emergency Medicine career, my medical practice, and my free medical clinic.

Does the literature back this up? Yes it does! This is known as the Faith Factor in health. There are many studies confirming this relationship between physical and spiritual health. A 1999 study on religious involvement and US mortality showed that those who never attended religious services had 1.87 times the risk of death as those who attend more than once weekly. This would result in a 7-year difference in life expectancy starting at age 20. In other words, those who go to church regularly live longer. And the longer you have done this, the greater the advantage.

Some people try to explain these findings by differences in lifestyle and diet. I don't agree. I have been going to church for years. I have watched what we serve at potluck gatherings and other church functions. Most of it is not a part of the recommendations we have discussed and is pretty unhealthy. The people don't look any thinner or take any extra precautions with their lifestyle. Some say this increased longevity is from the reduced stress from a sense of community and fellowship. There may be some truth to that. Clearly, the main reason, in my opinion, for this increased life expectancy is that God just chooses to bless those who obey Him. Its good to go to church for many reasons. Now, you can add physical health to the list.

Contrary to the media spin, Americans are still very interested in religion. According to the Pew Forum, 76% of US adults claim to be Christian. Of the remainder, 16% are unaffiliated, 4% are other religions, 1.6% are atheists and 2.4% are agnostics. 92% of Americans believe in God, but only 60% believe in a personal God. 63% believe the Bible is the Word of God. However, only 1/3 of Americans attend church in a given week. Clearly there is a disconnect between beliefs and behaviors in America.

When examining the mental health literature, participation in religious ceremonies, religious social support, prayer and personal significance of one's relationship with God were beneficial to mental health status 92% of the time. Frequent church attendance has been found to be protective against alcohol and drug abuse, suicide and delinquency in young people and adults. Why aren't mental health professionals addressing the spiritual needs of their patients? The problem is that numerous studies show that there is a tremendous lack of spirituality and religious attendance among mental health professionals.

Studies have documented the relationship between infrequent church attendance and physical health. The negative health effects include an increased incidence of Cardiovascular Disease, Hypertension, stroke and cancer. Going to church weekly has a positive effect on physical and mental health. Frequent church attendance was found to be protective. For example, those attending religious services weekly had a 5 mm Hg diastolic blood pressure (the bottom number) lower than those not going that often.

A 1988 prospective study of 4000 adults followed for 6 years showed something fascinating. Those attending religious services once a week or more, coupled with prayer and studying the Bible daily, had a 40% lower risk of Hypertension than those doing so less often. This was after controlling for other variables. There is a protective effect of going to church and reading your Bible regularly.

Spiritual conflicts and a lack of spiritual health clearly affect physical and mental health. Since the evidence of benefit is overwhelming, we should be encouraging our family, friends, patients, and co-workers to attend religious services at a Bible-believing church and to pray. We should be telling people the advantages of addressing their spiritual health and giving guidance on where to start.

Psalm 107:20 says, *He sent His word and healed them and delivered them from their destructions.* The Word of God is healing: physically, emotionally and spiritually. It sets people free from bondage and addictions. It helps people break them free from sins and habits that are destructive to them and others. Do you need to be healed of something? One of the names of God in the Old Testament is Jehovah-rapha, the Lord Who Heals. Let Him heal you using God's Word. It is the healing ointment, the balm of Gilead, we need to get well physically as well as spiritually.

Our God has given us great and mighty promises in His Word. These are not like the promises people make to you and then quickly beak them. How can you really trust them to keep their word after that? God's promises will never be broken. They are forever and He never changes. The universe and people change, but our God never changes. He is the same yesterday, today and forever. You can trust our God, YHWH, to keep His Word to you. Study His promises in Appendix 1 and refer to them often.

If you have read parts of the Bible before, why don't you try reading the whole thing? It is a great accomplishment to read the entire Bible. Very few people in the world have done that. There are good plans available for your phone and hard copy Bibles that you can purchase that divide up the Bible into 365 daily readings. Some come with a short devotion. When you read the whole Bible, you begin to see God's unfolding story for mankind and this world. You get a greater understanding of who God is and what He is like. You also come to understand what He wants for you.

Summary

We are in a health and healthcare crisis that no government can fix. Toxin exposures and nutrient deficiencies are ubiquitous, resulting in endless disease and the draining of financial resources. Poor lifestyle choices for the past 60 years have resulted in an epidemic of degenerative diseases and suffering. A medical establishment rooted in treating symptoms instead of the cause has left patients with a bag full of medications and no improvement in their health. Big pharaceutical, chemical and agriculture companies are making mountains of money at the expense of our health while the government that is supposed to protect us sits by and watches from the sidelines.

Individuals and families must adopt an **anti-inflammatory lifestyle** and take ownership of their health. We must stop relying on others to take care of us and pursue our own health and wellness. Knowledge is power. I have tried to provide you with a lot of information in this book. Now, you must choose to use it. There is a lot at stake for you and your families.

I have tried to stress the balancing of your body, mind, and spirit in this book. Each is important. Too much care of one without caring for the other parts leaves you still out of balance. Many people today are ignoring their spiritual life and focusing on physical health only. Remember, physical health is only of temporary benefit, in this life; without a vibrant relationship with God through Jesus Christ, this will be all there is. Jesus said in Matthew 6:33, *But seek first His kingdom and His righteousness, and all these things will be added to you.*

For those looking for a simple, get-started plan at this point, here are my Top 10 things to do right now to begin your journey to better health and a balanced life.

PFH Action Point: Top 10 things to do right now to get started

- **Eliminate wheat and dairy from your diet**
- **Eliminate sugars and processed foods from your diet**
- **Eat lots of fruits and vegetables in a rainbow of colors, preferably organic and raw**
- **Avoid all GMO foods, canned tuna (mercury, BPA) and rice products (arsenic)**
- **Stop drinking anything except reverse osmosis water and herbal teas that you make**
- **Get the plastic out of your kitchen and don't drink out of plastic containers**
- **Look for toxins in personal care products and eliminate them; use olive oil soap to start**
- **Check your vitamin D3 blood level and take supplements to get it to around 60**
- **Get 7-8 hours of quality sleep daily; use supplements if needed**
- **Address your spiritual health: start reading the Bible daily and get to know your Father in Heaven; claim God's Promises for you**

So what are you waiting for? Start your journey to better health today! Go back and read this book again. Take some notes this time. Find the areas you need to improve and make the changes that need to be made. Partner with your spouse or a friend and do this journey together. Determine to live a balanced life in our toxic world. This is your *Prescription for Health.*

Appendix 1

GOD'S PROMISES FOR YOU

By Alan W. Gruning, DO

Just think about this the next time you are feeling down, depressed, fearful, alone, anxious, or otherwise empty. While you were still lost, and not thinking about God at all, He was still thinking about you! He had a plan to save you, to set you free, and to give you a life of abundance and significance.

What follows are the promises from God's Word for you. *He sent His word and healed them and delivered them from their destructions.* (Psalm 107:20) Read them, look up the verses for yourself, review them often, and claim them as your own. Learn to replace the lies of the devil with the truth from God's Word.

1. **God knew you.** *For those whom He foreknew, He also predestined to become conformed to the image of His Son, so that He would be the firstborn among many brethren.* (Romans 8:29) God knew you when He created you, when He made you in your mother's womb. *I will give thanks to You, for I am fearfully and wonderfully made; wonderful are Your works, and my soul knows it very well.* Psalm 139:14 says you are fearfully and wonderfully made. You are a masterpiece, a special work of creative genius according to Ephesians 2:10. *For we are His workmanship, created in Christ Jesus for good works, which God prepared beforehand so that we would walk in them.* God knew you while you were growing up and when you became a teenager. God knew you when you were good and when you were bad. God knew you while you were running towards Him and running away from Him. He has seen everything you have ever done or thought, including all of the sins you have ever committed. And yet He still loves you.

2. God predestined you to become the image of His Son, Jesus. *For those whom He foreknew, He also predestined to become conformed to the image of His Son, so that He would be the firstborn among many brethren.* (Romans 8:29) That means He chose you to be His before you ever chose God. He did not have to choose you; He chose you because He wanted to, because of His great love for you. Believe it or not, you are very important to God, a one of a kind creation. And He wants you to become like Jesus.

3. God called you. *And these whom He predestined, He also called; and these whom He called, He also justified; and these whom He justified, He also glorified.* (Romans 8:30) This means you were sanctified, or set apart for His purpose. God called you out from the life you were living apart from Him and called you into a relationship with the Father. He did not have to do this. He did it because of His great mercy and love for you. He wants no one to perish, but all to come to eternal life. *The Lord is not slow about His promise, as some count slowness, but is patient toward you, not wishing for any to perish but for all to come to repentance.* (2 Peter 3:9)

4. The Father drew you to Jesus. *No one can come to Me unless the Father who sent Me draws him; and I will raise him up on the last day.* (John 6:44) There was still a problem. You did not care about God. You were still living your own life the way you wanted. The Father in Heaven had to draw you to Jesus. It was not your idea. It was His. Some people probably were praying for you. God heard and answered their prayers. If the Father had not drawn you to Jesus, you would still be lost. Why did God choose to draw you to Jesus? It is all about grace, the undeserved favor of God. You did not deserve it. His grace is greater than all your sins.

5. You were given the free gift of eternal life. The Bible says that we are all sinners. Romans 3:23 says *for all have sinned and fall short of the glory of God.* This means we do things and think things that are an offense to our holy God and violate his laws. Now, before you say that you are a pretty good person and not a bad sinner, let's take a look at God's standards, the 10 Commandments. Have you ever told a lie? What does that make you? A liar. Have you ever taken something that was not yours, even something little? That makes you a thief. Have you ever used the name of God or Jesus as a cuss word? That is called blasphemy. Have you ever looked with lust on a person that you were not married to? Jesus said that was as bad as committing adultery. Have you ever hated someone in your heart? Jesus said that was the same as murdering them. By all accounts, you are a lying thief, a blasphemer, adulterer, and murderer at heart. On Judgment Day, will you be guilty or innocent in the sight of God? Guilty as charged. You are a sinner.

For the wages of sin is death, but the free gift of God is eternal life in Christ Jesus our Lord. (Romans 6:23) The wages of our sins, or what we deserve to be paid for the sins we commit (in our actions *and* our thoughts), is death. This means eternal separation from God in a place called Hell, created for the devil and his rebellious angels, called demons. Our loving Father does not want any of His creation to go to Hell. Romans 5:8 says *But God demonstrates His own love toward us, in that while we were yet sinners, Christ died for us.* God sent His Son, Jesus, God in the flesh, to die on the cross in our place and give us the free gift of eternal life in Heaven. How do we get this free gift? Just by taking it! *For God so loved the world, that He gave His only begotten Son, that whoever believes in Him shall not perish, but have eternal life.* John 3:16 says that God so loved you that He gave His one and only Son, that if you believe in Jesus you will not perish, but you will have eternal life.

It is all about Jesus. It is not about you or how good you are. You are a sinner and not good at all. Isaiah 64:6 says, *For all of us have become like one who is unclean, and all our righteous deeds are like a filthy garment; and all of us wither like a leaf, and our iniquities, like the wind, take us away.* Your good deeds are like filthy rags to our holy God. You can't do enough good things to make up for all the sins you have committed in your life. You can't get the gift by being good. There is nothing you can do or pay to get it. It only comes by believing in Jesus and His death, burial and resurrection for you! It is truly a gift.

Ephesians 2:8-9 says, *For by grace you have been saved through faith; and that not of yourselves, it is the gift of God; not as a result of works, so that no one may boast.* If you could work you way to Heaven you would boast about how good you are. Salvation is by the grace of God alone. However, you have to choose to take this free gift. If you don't, then John 3:18 says that you are condemned to Hell because of *your* choice. *He who believes in Him is not judged; he who does not believe has been judged already, because he has not believed in the name of the only begotten Son of God.* It is that simple. Have you chosen to take the free gift of God?

6. **The veil was removed.** *But whenever a person turns to the Lord, the veil is taken away.* (2 Corinthians 3:16) The Father sent the Holy Spirit to intervene and convict you of your sins and your need for the Savior, Jesus. You decided to turn to the Lord Jesus. Whether it was a logical, controlled turning or you cried out in desperation because of the mess of your life, you chose to turn to Jesus. When you did, the Holy Spirit removed the covering that your enemy, Satan, had put over your eyes to blind you to the truth. Your eyes had been covered for many years. You had resisted every attempt He had made to reach you with the gospel, the good news. Thank the Lord that He did not give up on you. All of a sudden, you could finally see the truth.

7. **You were born again.** *Jesus answered and said to him, "Truly, truly, I say to you, unless one is born again he cannot see the kingdom of God."* (John 3:3) When you confessed your sins, asked for forgiveness, and agreed to turn from your sinful way of living (repentance) to become a follower of Jesus Christ and pursue holiness, you were saved. Romans 10:9-10 says *that if you confess with your mouth Jesus as Lord, and believe in your heart that God raised Him from the dead, you will be saved; for with the heart a person believes, resulting in righteousness, and with the mouth he confesses, resulting in salvation.* This means that you have to confess with your mouth that Jesus is your Lord and Savior, your Master and Owner, and that you have to give Him the control of your life as His servant and slave. You also have to believe in your heart that the Resurrection is true and Jesus is alive and will return as He promised.

And He was saying to them all, "If anyone wishes to come after Me, he must deny himself, and take up his cross daily and follow Me. For whoever wishes to save his life will lose it, but whoever loses his life for My sake, he is the one who will save it. Luke 9:23-24 says that if you want to be a follower of Jesus, you have to deny yourself, take up your cross daily and follow Him. That means you have to deny your agenda, plans, lusts, and desires and agree to live for Jesus. You have to carry your cross through the streets, publicly identifying with Jesus and not ashamed to follow Him. When you did these things, you were born again into the family of God. **If you have not done these things, you need to right now!** Otherwise, none of the rest of God's promises will apply to you. Just pray. God will hear your voice.

Jesus said in John 14:6, *I am the way, and the truth, and the life; no one comes to the Father but through Me.* You can only get to Heaven through Jesus. You can't get there by any other religion, person, beliefs, good works or anything you can do or pay. Do you believe that? Do you want His free gift of eternal life?

Here is a suggested prayer, to say out loud (confess with your mouth), if you want to be born again:

Father, thank You for loving me and never giving up on me. I confess I am a sinner and I want to repent of my sins and pursue holiness. Thank you Jesus for coming to this earth, dying on the cross, and shedding Your blood, for me. I give You the control of my life and want to follow You, Jesus. Make me into the Christian You want me to be. Thank You for saving me, Jesus. Amen.

Congratulations! If you prayed that prayer from your heart, you have been forgiven and born again into the family of God. The Holy Spirit has come to live in you. You have a home reserved in Heaven. You have peace with God.

8. **You were justified by faith**. *And these whom He predestined, He also called; and these whom He called, He also justified; and these whom He justified, He also glorified.* (Romans 8:30) When you gave your life to Jesus and trusted in His shed blood to save you, The Father justified you, making you holy and righteous in His sight. You could not enter Heaven in the sinful, filthy condition you were in. And there was nothing you

could do to make yourself righteous. Now, you have been washed clean and your sins forgiven by faith in Jesus Christ alone. This makes you able to spend eternity with the Father in Heaven. Once there, you will be glorified with a new body, perfect and eternal. Praise the Lord!

9. **Jesus Christ now lives in you.** *Test yourselves to see if you are in the faith; examine yourselves! Or do you not recognize this about yourselves, that Jesus Christ is in you—unless indeed you fail the test?* (2 Corinthians 13:5) When you are born again, Jesus comes to live in you. We are to test ourselves to see if we are in the faith. If Jesus lives in you, you will be different and want to live differently. Your goals and priorities will change to be more like His. You will want to do what He wants you to do. You will want to be what He wants you to be. Does that describe you?

10. **You have the Holy Spirit living in you.** *In Him, you also, after listening to the message of truth, the gospel of your salvation—having also believed, you were sealed in Him with the Holy Spirit of promise, who is given as a pledge of our inheritance, with a view to the redemption of God's own possession, to the praise of His glory.* (Ephesians 1:13-14) God has placed a seal on you that marks you as His child. The Holy Spirit is the deposit that guarantees your inheritance. The Holy Spirit is your Teacher, Counselor, Comforter and Helper. He will enable you to live the Christian life. You just need to cooperate with Him.

11. **You are a new creation.** *Therefore if anyone is in Christ, he is a new creature; the old things passed away; behold, new things have come.* (2 Corinthians 5:17) The old life is gone and forgotten by God. He has forgotten your sins. *As far as the east is from the west, so far has He removed our transgressions from us.* (Psalm 103:12) That means He remembers them no more. You are starting over, brand new in Jesus Christ. *Therefore there is now no condemnation for those who are in Christ Jesus.* (Romans 8:1) Because you are forgiven and made new, you should never feel condemned by God for your past. The devil wants you to feel condemned; he is a liar and the father of lies. Don't listen to him. Listen to Jesus. The truth will set you free.

12. **You are adopted into God's family.** *For you have not received a spirit of slavery leading to fear again, but you have received a spirit of adoption as sons by which we cry out, "Abba! Father!"* (Romans 8:15) *For you are all sons of God through faith in Christ Jesus.* (Galatians 3:26) God is now your Father and you are now His son or daughter, with all the rights and privileges of a family member. You can come to Him at any time and call Him "Abba" (daddy) and "Father." You can sit in His lap, enjoy His company, and talk to Him about anything. Think of it, the God who created everything wants to have that kind of relationship with you.

13. **You are an heir.** *And if children, heirs also, heirs of God and fellow heirs with Christ, if indeed we suffer with Him so that we may also be glorified with Him.* (Romans 8:17) You will inherit a great fortune. You are a co-heir with Christ of all of Heaven. All that the Father has created in Heaven is there for your enjoyment. We can't begin to imagine all that the Father has for us there.

14. **You are seated in Heaven with Christ.** *And raised us up with Him, and seated us with Him in the heavenly places in Christ Jesus.* (Ephesians 2:6) Your home is now in Heaven and you are just visiting here on earth. Since Christ is seated on His throne, you are seated with Him on a throne.

15. **You have crowns.** *In the future there is laid up for me the crown of righteousness, which the Lord, the righteous Judge, will award to me on that day; and not only to me, but also to all who have loved His appearing.* 2 Timothy 4:8 says you have been given a crown of righteousness. *Blessed is a man who perseveres under trial; for once he has been approved, he will receive the crown of life which the Lord has promised to those who love Him.* (James 1:12) *Do not fear what you are about to suffer. Behold, the devil is about to cast some of you into prison, so that you will be tested, and you will have tribulation for ten days. Be faithful until death, and I will give you the crown of life.* (Revelation 2:10) Faithful followers have been given the crown of life. *And when the Chief Shepherd appears, you will receive the unfading crown of glory.* 1 Peter 5:4 says believers have been given the crown of glory. Instead of the crown of thorns that Jesus wore for you

on the earth, you have been given golden crowns that you will wear in Heaven and will lay at His feet.

16. **You are more than a conqueror.** *But in all these things we overwhelmingly conquer through Him who loved us.* (Romans 8:37) Through Christ, you can now conquer anything, including the devil, temptation, sin, habits, and evil. *But thanks be to God, who always leads us in triumph in Christ, and manifests through us the sweet aroma of the knowledge of Him in every place.* 2 Corinthians 2:14 says that God leads us in triumph in Christ.

17. **You can resist temptation and sin.** *No temptation has overtaken you but such as is common to man; and God is faithful, who will not allow you to be tempted beyond what you are able, but with the temptation will provide the way of escape also, so that you will be able to endure it.* (1 Corinthians 10:13) The Holy Spirit has given you the ability to resist temptation. You can exercise self-control, which is the exercise of inner strength, under the direction of sound judgment, which enables us to do, think, and say the things that are pleasing to God. This may mean getting rid of the things that tempt you to sin, such as old friends, places you go, things you watch on TV or the internet, or things you read. It also means filling yourself with the things of God that will build up your spirit, such as reading the Bible daily, going to church, finding some Christian friends, watching Christian TV, listening to Christian music, etc. Remember, the battlefield is in the mind. Stop the thoughts before they enter your mind or you dwell on them. Thoughts lead to actions.

18. **You can live a holy life.** *Pursue peace with all men, and the sanctification without which no one will see the Lord.* (Hebrews 12:14) You are to pursue peace and sanctification (holiness). In fact, without holiness, no one will see the Lord! This is not an option to our holy God. He expects us to pursue a holy life. You have the Spirit of God living inside you and He has given you the ability to live a holy life. It is all about your obedience to the revealed will of God. You just have to cooperate with Him. As we covered above, He will give you the strength to resist temptation and sin. You just have to ask for His help.

19. **You can do all things.** *I can do all things through Him who strengthens me.* (Philippians 4:13) Through Christ, everything is now possible for you to accomplish, not in your strength, but in His. In 2 Corinthians 12:9-10, God tells Paul that His grace is sufficient for every need we have. *And He has said to me, "My grace is sufficient for you, for power is perfected in weakness." Most gladly, therefore, I will rather boast about my weaknesses, so that the power of Christ may dwell in me. Therefore I am well content with weaknesses, with insults, with distresses, with persecutions, with difficulties, for Christ's sake; for when I am weak, then I am strong.* He says that His power is made perfect in our weakness. So, Paul concludes that when we are weak, that is when we are strong because of God's power.

20. **God will supply all your needs.** *And my God will supply all your needs according to His riches in glory in Christ Jesus.* (Philippians 4:19) You don't have to worry or be anxious about anything you need. God will supply it according to His riches in glory in Christ Jesus. God owns it all and has unlimited access to resources for you. Note this does not include your wants, but your needs.

21. **You will never be hungry or thirsty again.** *Jesus said to them, "I am the bread of life; he who comes to Me will not hunger, and he who believes in Me will never thirst.* (John 6:35) Jesus said that He was the bread of life and that whoever came to Him would no longer be hungry and whoever believed in Him would no longer be thirsty. This is true both in the physical realm and the spiritual realm.

22. **You can approach God boldly.** *Therefore let us draw near with confidence to the throne of grace, so that we may receive mercy and find grace to help in time of need.* (Hebrews 4:16) As God's son or daughter, you can feel confident to approach the Father on His throne of grace at any time with any need. You will receive mercy and find grace to help in your time of need.

23. **You can ask for anything.** *This is the confidence which we have before Him, that, if we ask anything according to His will, He hears us. And if we know that He hears us in whatever we ask, we know that we have the requests which we have asked from Him.* (1 John 5:14-15) If you ask for

anything according to God's will, He hears your request and you will have what you asked for. If it is not God's will, you won't receive your request because it is probably not good for you or the wrong timing.

24. Jesus is your intercessor. *Therefore He is able also to save forever those who draw near to God through Him, since He always lives to make intercession for them.* (Hebrews 7:25) Jesus takes your requests and needs and goes to the Father on your behalf. That is why we are instructed to pray in the name of Jesus. *If you ask Me anything in My name, I will do it.* (John 14:14)

25. God is working all things out for your good. *And we know that God causes all things to work together for good to those who love God, to those who are called according to His purpose.*)Romans 8:28) The Father, Son, and Holy Spirit are looking at every situation in your life and working things out for your good, <u>if</u> you love the Lord and have been called to His purpose. The Father and Son send ministering angels to help and guide you. The Holy Spirit of God lives in you and shows you the right path to be on.

26. God's plans are to give you hope and a future. *For I know the plans that I have for you, declares the Lord, plans for welfare and not for calamity, to give you a future and a hope.* (Jeremiah 29:11) The Father wants only good things for you. He has plans for your life. His plans are to prosper you, not to harm you. He wants to give you a future full of hope knowing that He is with you.

27. You have a mansion in Heaven. *In My Father's house are many dwelling places; if it were not so, I would have told you; for I go to prepare a place for you.* (John 14:2) Based on the description of the New Jerusalem in Revelation, scholars have estimated that your home there is perhaps 10,000 square feet-a mansion! There will be no bad views and you will not have to clean it since there is no dirt or dust.

28. Jesus will return to take you to Heaven. *If I go and prepare a place for you, I will come again and receive you to Myself, that where I am, there you may be also.* (John 14:3) *For the Lord Himself will descend from heaven with a shout, with the voice of the archangel and with the trumpet* *of God, and the dead in Christ will rise first. Then we who are alive and remain will be caught up together with them in the clouds to meet the Lord in the air, and so we shall always be with the Lord. Therefore comfort one another with these words.* (1 Thessalonians 4:16-18) Jesus promised He would return and take you to the Father's house. Know the signs of the times. We are living in the last days. His return is very near.

29. **You will have a new body, perfect, like Jesus Christ.** *Behold, I tell you a mystery; we will not all sleep, but we will all be changed, in a moment, in the twinkling of an eye, at the last trumpet; for the trumpet will sound, and the dead will be raised imperishable, and we will be changed. For this perishable must put on the imperishable, and this mortal must put on immortality.* (1 Corinthians 15:51-53) *Who will transform the body of our humble state into conformity with the body of His glory, by the exertion of the power that He has even to subject all things to Himself.* (Philippians 3:21) Our eternal body in Heaven will be without pain, disease, flaws, and any imperfections. Some believe we will be 33 years old, like Jesus at His death. We will be able to transport anywhere in the universe instantaneously and pass through objects like Jesus did. I can't wait for the new body I was promised!

30. **Jesus has given you an abundant life now.** *The thief comes only to steal and kill and destroy; I came that they may have life, and have it abundantly.* (John 10:10) You don't have to wait for Heaven to experience the peace, joy, and purpose God has for you.

31. **Jesus will never leave you or forsake you.** *Make sure that your character is free from the love of money, being content with what you have; for He Himself has said, "I will never desert you, nor will I ever forsake you."* (Hebrews 13:5) You are never alone. Jehovah-shammah (The Lord is there) is always with you. In fact, the Holy Spirit of the living God lives inside of you! He is with you in the good times and the bad. He is with you when you are being persecuted or suffering for the Name of Jesus. He is with you when people hurt you and you are brokenhearted. He is with you when nothing seems to be going right and your world is falling apart. Jesus understands the pain you are going through. He went through all these things, too. He did it all for you.

32. **God will direct your life and lead you on the right path.** *Your ears will hear a word behind you, 'This is the way, walk in it,' whenever you turn to the right or to the left.* (Isaiah 30:21) *Thus says the Lord, your Redeemer, the Holy One of Israel, 'I am the Lord your God, who teaches you to profit, Who leads you in the way you should go.'* (Isaiah 48:17) You will hear God's voice and experience the counsel and help of the Holy Spirit as you make decisions about what path and direction to take. However, you must spend time to listen to His voice and want to hear it. We live in a time of great distraction and busyness. You need to turn off all those distractions for a time daily and spend a Quiet Time with your Father in order to hear His voice. Just read the Bible and pray, talking to God. Take the time to listen throughout the day to the Holy Spirit speaking to you.

33. **God will renew your strength.** *Yet those who wait for the Lord Will gain new strength; they will mount up with wings like eagles, they will run and not get tired, they will walk and not become weary.*

(Isaiah 40:31) If you wait for the Lord, He will strengthen you for the challenges and trials ahead. You can mount up with wings like eagles. You will run and not get tired. You will walk and not get weary.

34. **The Holy Spirit is your Helper.** *But the Helper, the Holy Spirit, whom the Father will send in My name, He will teach you all things, and bring to your remembrance all that I said to you.* (John 14:26) You do not have to do life alone. He will help you make the right decisions and keep you on the right path.

35. **You have been filled with the fruits of the Spirit.** *But the fruit of the Spirit is love, joy, peace, patience, kindness, goodness, faithfulness, gentleness, and self-control; against such things there is no law.* (Galatians 5:22) You have been given love, joy, peace, patience, kindness, goodness, faithfulness, gentleness (and humility), and self-control. These are not natural qualities. They have been given to you so that people will see Jesus in you.

36. **You have been given spiritual gifts.** *But to each one is given the manifestation of the Spirit for the common good.* (1 Corinthians 12:7)

They are supernatural and special gifts from God, just for you. With these gifts, you will build up the church and help other believers.

37. **You are a part of Christ's body.** *Now you are Christ's body, and individually members of it.* (1 Corinthians 12:27) His body is the church. You are an important part of it. You make it healthy and work right.

38. **You can be wise.** *But if any of you lacks wisdom, let him ask of God, who gives to all generously and without reproach, and it will be given to him.* (James 1:5) You can ask for wisdom from God and He will give it to you. Then, you will know what to do and what decisions to make. *The fear of the Lord is the beginning of wisdom, and the knowledge of the Holy One is understanding.* (Proverbs 9:10) Fear means awe, reverence, respect and willing submission to the God who made you and everything else. You can't be wise until you first understand the fear of the LORD and learn as much as possible about Him. That comes from reading His Word, the Bible, and spending time with Him.

39. **You have been given work to do.** *For we are His workmanship, created in Christ Jesus for good works, which God prepared beforehand so that we would walk in them.* (Ephesians 2:10) You were created to accomplish important things. You have a purpose in this life. *Who has saved us and called us with a holy calling, not according to our works, but according to His own purpose and grace which was granted us in Christ Jesus from all eternity.* 2 Timothy 1:9 says you have been given a holy calling. You are to do good works, not as a way to earn salvation and approval from God. He cannot love you more than He already does. You are to do good works because it is your way to give back to the Lord for all He has done for you.

40. **You have peace.** *Peace I leave with you; My peace I give to you; not as the world gives do I give to you. Do not let your heart be troubled, nor let it be fearful.* (John 14:27) Jesus has given you peace. The world does not give you peace, only stress. In Jesus, you have real peace with God and the security of His love and your home in Heaven. Nothing else really matters.

41. **You have freedom from anxiety.** *Be anxious for nothing, but in everything by prayer and supplication with thanksgiving let your requests be made known to God. And the peace of God, which surpasses all comprehension, will guard your hearts and your minds in Christ Jesus.* (Philippians 4:6-7) You do not have to be anxious about anything. In fact, you are commanded not to be. Instead, you are to pray, bringing your requests to God, and be thankful for what you do have instead of worried about what you don't have. The peace of God will guard your heart and mind in Christ Jesus.

42. **You have victory.** *Submit therefore to God. Resist the devil and he will flee from you.* (James 4:7) If you submit to God's will and His Word, and resist the devil, he will flee from you. Remember, you are more than a conqueror through Christ. Take authority over the devil. Command him to leave (out loud-he can't read your thoughts). You are holy ground. *Put on the full armor of God, so that you will be able to stand firm against the schemes of the devil. For our struggle is not against flesh and blood, but against the rulers, against the powers, against the world forces of this darkness, against the spiritual forces of wickedness in the heavenly places.* (Ephesians 6:11-12) God has given you weapons to use against the devil and his lies. Learn about them and use them in Ephesians 6:14-17.

43. **You are healed.** *But He was pierced through for our transgressions, He was crushed for our iniquities; the chastening for our well-being fell upon Him, and by His scourging we are healed. All of us like sheep have gone astray, each of us has turned to his own way; but the Lord has caused the iniquity of us all to fall on Him.* (Isaiah 53:5-6) By the stripes of Jesus, you have been healed. That means physically, emotionally, and spiritually.

44. **You can rest.** *The Lord is my shepherd, I shall not want. He makes me lie down in green pastures; He leads me beside quiet waters. He restores my soul; He guides me in the paths of righteousness For His name's sake.* (Psalm 23:1-3) The Lord, your Shepherd, takes care of all your needs. So, you can lie down and rest in perfect peace. You can drink from the living water He provides. You can be at peace knowing that He restores you when you fall down from sin. He will lead you in the right path, the one that leads to righteousness, not the one the rest of

the world is on that leads to destruction. You belong to Him and He cares for your every need.

45. **You have nothing to fear.** *Even though I walk through the valley of the shadow of death, I fear no evil, for You are with me; Your rod and Your staff, they comfort me.* (Psalm 23:4) Jesus is walking with you through the valleys of life and leads you to the mountaintops. He has a rod (the Bible) and a staff (the Holy Spirit) to comfort you and protect you from predators. When you stray away, He brings you back. However, He also will discipline you when you do wrong. *For those whom the Lord loves He disciplines, and He scourges every son whom He receives.* (Hebrews 12:6) *For they disciplined us for a short time as seemed best to them, but He disciplines us for our good, so that we may share His holiness.* (Hebrews 12:10) Discipline is for your good because the Father disciplines those He loves like a parent so that we will grow to become more like Jesus.

46. **You can experience God's abundance and care.** *You prepare a table before me in the presence of my enemies; You have anointed my head with oil; my cup overflows.* (Psalm 23:5) The Good Shepherd has prepared an abundant table for you full of good things and free of harmful things. This is in full sight of your enemies, the enemies of God. Hopefully, they will see what the Lord is doing in your life and want the same! He anoints your head with the oil of the Holy Spirit to cure you of the devil's temptations and lies that try to creep into your mind and scar your life. He also frees you from the need to fight with others for your rights since He takes care of all your needs anyway. Truly, your cup runs over with His provision.

47. **You can be secure in God's love for you.** *Surely goodness and lovingkindness will follow me all the days of my life, and I will dwell in the house of the Lord forever.* (Psalm 23:6) Goodness and loving kindness will follow you all the days of your life. You will dwell in the house of the Lord forever. Nothing will ever change that. Romans 8:38-39 says *For I am convinced that neither death, nor life, nor angels, nor principalities, nor things present, nor things to come, nor powers, nor height, nor depth,*

nor any other created thing, will be able to separate us from the love of God, which is in Christ Jesus our Lord. What a promise!

48. You will see God's face and His Name will be on your forehead. *They will see His face, and His name will be on their foreheads.* (Revelation 22:4) In the Old Testament, no one could look on God's face and live. You will see God face to face, just as His friend Moses did. And you will belong to the Lord forever as His treasured possession.

49. You can be an overcomer. Revelation 3 is full of God's promises to those who overcome the evils of this world and resist the devil. You will eat of the tree of life in the Paradise of God. You will not be hurt by the second death. You will be given hidden manna, the bread of God, and a new name from the Lord. You will be given authority to rule over the nations with Jesus. You will be given white garments, your name will not be erased from the Book of Life, and Jesus will confess you as His follower before His Father and the angels. You will be a pillar in the temple of God in Heaven and Jesus will write the Name of God on you. You will sit with Jesus on His throne in Heaven. *He who overcomes will inherit these things, and I will be his God and he will be My son.* Revelation 21:7 says that he who overcomes will inherit all God's blessings mentioned and God will be your God and you will be His son or daughter forever.

50. You can come to the Lord. *The Spirit and the bride say, "Come." And let the one who hears say, "Come." And let the one who is thirsty come; let the one who wishes take the water of life without cost.* (Revelation 22:17) The Spirit and the bride say, "Come." You can come and drink from the water of life without cost. It is free. You have heard God's promises for His people. Are you one of His elect? You can be. Review #7 above. If you have not surrendered the control of your life to Jesus Christ, do it now. You have nothing to lose and all of Heaven and eternity to gain. It is your choice. However, remember, no choice is a choice. Choose life and the promises God has for you!

I hope these promises have left you feeling loved, special, and at peace. Review them often. Thank the Lord for His Word to you. Choose to live for Him.

CPSIA information can be obtained
at www.ICGtesting.com
Printed in the USA
FFOW01n1604030618
46992658-49261FF